RECENT ADVANCES IN HEMATOLOGY RESEARCH

SICKLE CELL DISEASE

GENETICS, MANAGEMENT AND PROGNOSIS

RECENT ADVANCES IN HEMATOLOGY RESEARCH

Additional books in this series can be found on Nova's website under the Series tab.

Additional e-books in this series can be found on Nova's website under the e-book tab.

RECENT ADVANCES IN HEMATOLOGY RESEARCH

SICKLE CELL DISEASE

GENETICS, MANAGEMENT AND PROGNOSIS

RECENT ADVANCES IN HEMATOLOGY RESEARCH

Additional books in this series can be found on Nova's website under the Series tab.

Additional e-books in this series can be found on Nova's website under the e-book tab.

RECENT ADVANCES IN HEMATOLOGY RESEARCH

SICKLE CELL DISEASE

GENETICS, MANAGEMENT AND PROGNOSIS

MARILYN E. LEWIS
EDITOR

NOVA BIOMEDICAL
New York

Library of Congress Cataloging-in-Publication Data

ISBN: 978-1-63482-828-4

Library of Congress Control Number: 2015939097

Published by Nova Science Publishers, Inc. † New York

Contents

Preface

Sickle cell disease (SCD) is a genetic disorder caused by an abnormality of hemoglobin. The disease is characterized by a chronic hemolytic anemia. The search for affordable and accessible medicines mainly from plants and having various modes of actions for managing SCD is a priority in Africa where the disease is endemic. The first chapter in this book reviews children with Sickle Cell Disease (SCD). The authors also present their research that shows that clinically, children with SCD behave differently regarding their genetics. The second chapter gives an overview of the current progress in research in calcium handling in red blood cells of sickle cell disease patients, followed by an outlook into the potential use of blockers of the cation channels for therapy of SCD patients. The third chapter reviews and validates the pharmacological relevance of "Gardenia ternifolia" and sustains the use of this herbal medicine in the management of SCD in traditional medical systems. The fourth chapter reviews the search and the development of antisickling herbal drugs in Africa, where Sickle cell disease (SCD) is an endemic. The last chapter reviews SCD and its impact on sexual functioning as well as relationship dynamics. Conclusions support the importance of social support and its far-reaching impact into the coping mechanisms of patients with chronic illness as well as quality of life.

Chapter I – Children and adolescents with Sickle Cell Disease (SCD) usually have a disturbed sleep comparing to controls without SCD. Usually they present a lower O2 saturation than other children with the same severity of obstructive sleep apnea (OSA) but without SCD. Clinically, children with SCD behave differently regarding their genetics, since some haplotypes seem to have more serious clinical complications such as stroke and acute chest syndrome. The presence of alpha-globin deletion and higher levels of fetal hemoglobin (HbF) modifies red cell indices and rheology, and positively influence clinical events. In Portugal, children with SCD are mainly born in families that came from Angola, Cape Verde and Guiné-Bissau so the most common haplotypes are Bantu, Benin and Senegal. Objectives: To describe polysomnographic sleep characteristics in a sample of children and adolescents with sickle cell disease that were previously studied regarding S haplotype, presence of alpha thalassemia and HbF basal level. Methods: This was a retrospective study that included 54 children and adolescents with SCD, aged 1 - 18 years previously submitted to a genetic characterization (S haplotype and alpha globin), and Hemoglobin F basal level determination. Subjects were divided in 2 age groups (1-8 and 9-18 years) regarding lymphoid tissue hypertrophy and adenotonsillectomy status. Considering their haplotype, alpha deletion and HbF level, sleep characteristics were studied namely efficiency, latency and REM latency and sleep phases percentage (N1, N2, N3 and REM), AHI index, SpO2 mean and minimum. Descriptive and nonparametric statistics were used. Results: From a sample of 54 children and adolescents , 55.6% male, aged mean 9.52 years (1-18Y) s.d. 4.1 with SCD, 2 groups were formed: group A, n= 21 (1-8Y), age mean 5.24; s.d. 1.78Y, 57.1% male and group B, n= 33 (9-18Y), age mean 12.24 , s.d. 2.48Y , male 54.5%. Regarding haplotype determination, Bantu/Bantu was predominant, 57.4% of subjects (group A-66.7%; group B-51.5%), and 42.5 % had alpha deletion mostly 3.7 deletion. Regarding HbF basal level, 21 individuals (38.9%) had HbF >10%. Presence of alpha deletion showed no influence in sleep characteristics including AHI and SpO2 mean and minimum. Instead, presence of HbF greater than 10% seems to be protective regarding AHI ($p<0.01$) in group B (older). Regarding respiratory parameters, OSA existed in 92.5 % of subjects with mean AIH 3.5/h, s.d 1.73 (0.4-9.5/h), SpO2 mean was 94.6%, s.d. 3.05 (87-99%) and SpO2 minimum mean was 90.0%, s.d. 5.37 (72-97%); 8 subjects had previously adenotonsillectomy (1 in group A; 7 in group B). Polysomnographic parameters were similar in all the haplotypes, finding no relevance in HbF level or thalassemic status. Conclusions: Although sleep is disturbed in children and adolescents with SCD compared with controls, haplotype does not seem to influence sleep characteristics. Instead, the presence of high levels of HbF seems to be protective regarding respiratory sleep disturbances, mainly AHI in older subjects with less adenoid and tonsils hypertrophy.

Chapter II – Precise control over the intracellular free Ca^{2+} level is of key importance for any cell, red blood cells (RBCs) included. Cell fate of erythroid precursor cells, as well as volume, redox state, deformability, aggregability, adherence to the endothelial layer, and membrane stability of circulating RBCs, and as a result RBC longevity, are regulated by Ca^{2+}. Several hereditary forms of hemolytic anemia, including sickle cell disease (SCD), are associated with abnormally high Ca^{2+} uptake, and as a result, Ca^{2+} overload. Multiple organ failure, stroke, and myocardial infarction caused by thrombosis as well as repeated hemolytic and pain crises are induced by irreversible polymerization of deoxygenated hemoglobin S in RBCs of these patients. Dehydration of RBCs speed up sickle cell transformation, extensive oxidation and facilitated proteolysis, as well as increased adherence of circulating RBCs to the endothelial layer, substantially contribute to the sickle cell disease manifestation. As all of these processes are driven by the high intraerythrocytic Ca^{2+} levels, inhibition of pathologically high Ca^{2+} uptake would be a powerful therapeutic strategy. Molecular identity of ion channels involved in pathologically high permeability of RBC membranes of patients for Ca^{2+} is a subject of intensive investigation. Among the identified channels are Piezo channels and N-methyl D-aspartate (NMDA) receptors. The contribution of transient voltage receptor channels (TRPCs), voltage-gated calcium channels Cav2.1, and even voltage-dependent anion channels (VDACs) into the Ca^{2+} uptake is currently being debated. This chapter is an overview of the current progress in research in this area followed by an outlook into the potential use of blockers of the cation channels for therapy of SCD patients.

Chapter III – *Background*: Sickle cell disease (SCD) is a genetic disorder caused by an abnormality of hemoglobin. The disease is characterized by a chronic hemolytic anemia. The search for affordable and accessible medicines mainly from plants and having various modes of actions for managing SCD is a priority in Africa where the disease is endemic. *Materials and Methods*: The antioxidant activity of crude extracts of *Gardenia jovis tonantis* leaves was carried out using DPPH free radical scavenging assay while *in vitro* antisickling activity was assessed on sickle erythrocytes by the Emmel's test as previously reported. *Results and Discussion*: Methanol soluble fraction, ethyl acetate soluble fraction and anthocyanin crude extracts displayed interesting *in vitro* radical scavenging and antisickling activities. These results confirm those already given by our research team with anthocyanins from other Congolese medicinal plants traditionally used in folk medicine for the management of SCD. As reducing agent/drug, anthocyanins based medicine could prevent *in vivo* oxidative reactions, often by scavenging free radicals before they can damage cells. *Conclusion*: This study has validated the pharmacological relevance of *Gardenia ternifolia* and sustains the use of this herbal medicine in the management of SCD in traditional medical system.

Chapter IV – Background: The search and the development of antisickling herbal drugs are a priority in Africa, where the Sickle cell disease (SCD) is endemic. The author's research program had as initial objectives - to identify plants traditionally used in folk medicine for the management of SCD in Democratic Republic of the Congo (DRC), - to identify other/new sources of antisickling bioactive secondary metabolites mainly from non human primate (great apes) pharmacopeia/diet or zoopharmacognosy - to validate their bioactivity scientifically, - to identify the chemical groups responsible for this bioactivity, to elucidate the structures the bioactive molecules and finally - to formulate the bioactive plants based medicines for managing SCD in DRC. Study design and Methodology: The plant extracts were screened for antisickling activity using Emmel test, polymerization of haemoglobin S assay; osmotic fragility assay; anti-hemolytic test; radical scavenging assay and Met-hemoglobin profiling assay. The molecular structures of the active compounds were characterized by combining the chromatographic and spectroscopic methods. The acute toxicity bioassay of herbal medicine was carried out using the Wistar rats as animal model. Results: To date, 100 antisickling plants were scientifically validated; - the anthocyanins, betulinic, maslinic, oleanolic and lunularic acid as well as the butyl stearate are responsible for this bioactivity. The results of the pre-clinical evaluations allowed us to select by bio-guidance three most active plants for the formulation of a polyherbal medicine Drepanoalpha®. This herbal drug displayed *in vitro* sickling inhibitory of effect on drepanocytes in hypoxia as well anti-hemolytic and anti-oxidative properties. The acute toxicity test in Wistar rat model showed that the DL_{50} of Drepanoalpha® is higher than 4000 mg/kg. The analysis of the biochemical and hematologic markers showed the safety of Drepanoalpha®. Thus, Drepanoalpha® is not toxic and has moreover the property of boosting the rate of hemoglobin in the treated rats. A preliminary clinical trial of Drepanoalpha® in a pilot scale on a sample of 20 sicklers indicates that this drug alleviate significantly clinical manifestations in patients after some period probably by epigenetic modulation of the gene expression of fetal hemoglobin or by inhibiting *in vivo* hemolysis of sickle erythrocytes. Non-recourse to blood transfusion is done for a long period after cessation of medication. Conclusion and future directions: The results of fundamental research obtained led us to develop Drepanoalpha® from Congolese Traditional Medicine knowledge. The biochemical and hematological data showed that this polyherbal formula does not interfere with the physiological functions of the liver and the kidneys. A double blind and randomized clinical trial (Phase II), is thus necessary for confirming the in vivo biosafety of the medicine before it industrial valorization.

Chapter V – Sickle Cell Disease (SCD) and other chronic diseases can certainly have a significant impact on sexual functioning as well as relationship dynamics, especially with the importance of support systems within the framework of a chronic illness. The sample consisted of 140 Jamaican adults between the ages of 19 and 79 years (mean age = 35.97 ± 12.11 years). Diagnosis of SCD was based on results of hemoglobin electrophoresis. Correlations were conducted with types of SCD pain, intensity of pain, sexual activity and social support from spouse with special attention paid to the emotional, instrumental, informational and comparison aspects of social support from the patient's spouse/significant other. Various questions regarding sexual functioning were utilized to explore this area. Results indicated that there were a number of significant correlations between sexual activity and support, pain and support, pain and quality of intimate relationship, spouse's reaction to pain and patient's pain ($p < .05$). Conclusions support the importance of social support and its far-reaching impact into the coping mechanisms of patients with chronic illness as well as quality of life.

In: Sickle Cell Disease
Editor: Marilyn E. Lewis
ISBN: 978-1-63482-828-4

Chapter I

Sickle Cell Disease-Genetics and Sleep

Helena Cristina Loureiro*[1,2,3]*, Alexandra Dias*[1,2]*,
***Maria Inês Mascarenhas*[1,2] *and Teresa Ferreira*[1,2]**
[1]Pediatric Department, Hospital Prof. Doutor Fernando Fonseca, Amadora, Portugal
[2]Sickle Cell Disease Pediatric Group, Pediatric Department, Hospital Prof. Doutor Fernando Fonseca, Amadora, Portugal
[3]Pediatric Sleep Laboratory, Hospital Prof. Doutor Fernando Fonseca, Amadora, Portugal

Abstract

Children and adolescents with Sickle Cell Disease (SCD) usually have a disturbed sleep comparing to controls without SCD. Usually they present a lower O2 saturation than other children with the same severity of obstructive sleep apnea (OSA) but without SCD. Clinically, children with SCD behave differently regarding their genetics, since some haplotypes seem to have more serious clinical complications such as stroke and acute chest syndrome.

The presence of alpha-globin deletion and higher levels of fetal hemoglobin (HbF) modifies red cell indices and rheology, and positively influence clinical events. In Portugal, children with SCD are mainly born in families that came from Angola, Cape Verde and Guiné-Bissau so the most common haplotypes are Bantu, Benin and Senegal.

Objectives: To describe polysomnographic sleep characteristics in a sample of children and adolescents with sickle cell disease that were previously studied regarding S haplotype, presence of alpha thalassemia and HbF basal level.

Methods: This was a retrospective study that included 54 children and adolescents with SCD, aged 1 - 18 years previously submitted to a genetic characterization (S haplotype and alpha globin), and Hemoglobin F basal level determination. Subjects were divided in 2 age groups (1-8 and 9-18 years) regarding lymphoid tissue hypertrophy and adenotonsillectomy status. Considering their haplotype, alpha deletion and HbF level, sleep characteristics were studied namely efficiency, latency and REM latency and sleep phases percentage (N1, N2, N3 and REM), AHI index, SpO2 mean and minimum. Descriptive and nonparametric statistics were used.

Results: From a sample of 54 children and adolescents , 55.6% male, aged mean 9.52 years (1-18Y) s.d. 4.1 with SCD, 2 groups were formed: group A, n= 21 (1-8Y), age mean 5.24; s.d. 1.78Y, 57.1% male and group B, n= 33 (9-18Y), age mean 12.24 , s.d. 2.48Y , male 54.5%. Regarding haplotype determination, Bantu/Bantu was predominant, 57.4% of subjects (group A-66.7%; group B-51.5%), and 42.5 % had alpha deletion mostly 3.7 deletion. Regarding HbF basal level, 21 individuals (38.9%) had HbF >10%. Presence of alpha deletion showed no influence in sleep characteristics including AHI and SpO2 mean and minimum. Instead, presence of HbF greater than 10% seems to be protective regarding AHI ($p<0.01$) in group B (older). Regarding respiratory parameters, OSA existed in 92.5 % of subjects with mean AIH 3.5/h, s.d 1.73 (0.4-9.5/h), SpO2 mean was 94.6%, s.d. 3.05 (87-99%) and SpO2 minimum mean was 90.0%, s.d. 5.37 (72-97%); 8 subjects had previously adenotonsillectomy (1 in group A; 7 in group B). Polysomnographic parameters were similar in all the haplotypes, finding no relevance in HbF level or thalassemic status.

Conclusions: Although sleep is disturbed in children and adolescents with SCD compared with controls, haplotype does not seem to influence sleep characteristics. Instead, the presence of high levels of HbF seems to be protective regarding respiratory sleep disturbances, mainly AHI in older subjects with less adenoid and tonsils hypertrophy.

Introduction

Sickle Cell Anemia is an inherited recessive blood disorder that affects millions of people, in different parts of the world, causing significant morbidity and mortality. Sickle cell disease is among the most common monogenetic diseases worldwide. It is estimated that 312,000 people with hemoglobin SS (Hb SS) are born each year throughout the world, with the majority of these births (236,000) in sub-Saharan Africa. Based on the World Health Organization published global prevalence map of SCD and other data [1] about 20–25 million individuals world-wide have homozygous SCD; 12–15 million in sub-Saharan Africa, 5–10 million in India and about 3 million distributed in other parts of the world. Migration patterns have led to the distribution of the sickle cell genes into regions that are not endemic for malaria.

Homozygous sickle cell disease is a chronic disorder in which a gene mutation (a single nucleotide change, GAG GTG, in the beta chain globin gene, and valine replaces glutamic acid at the sixth amino acid position in the beta globin chain) leads to an abnormal globin protein and to the formation of a functional different hemoglobin molecule (hemoglobin S): although retaining the capacity to carry oxygen, after deoxygenating easily polymerizes, inducing the red cell shape and rigidity changes, leading to serious pathologic consequences [2]. Vaso-occlusion and hemolysis related to these rigid and/or sickled cells lead to disease manifestations, including hemolytic anemia, severe pain episodes from bone marrow ischemia, central nervous system strokes, the acute chest syndrome, pulmonary hypertension, left-sided heart disease, bacteremia, leg ulcers, growth failure, priapism and damage to the spleen, kidneys, liver and bones.

Although these individuals are homozygous to Hb S, they exhibit a large diversity in clinical and laboratory phenotypes. This heterogeneity is evidenced also in the severe outcomes such as stroke, acute chest syndrome, avascular necrosis and other painful vaso-occlusive episodes, and is related to genetic modifiers and environmental effects. Clinically, children and adolescents with SCD behave differently regarding their genetics, hematologic or other (like UDP-glucuronosyl transferase 1A1 gene promoter polymorphisms); some haplotypes seem to have more serious clinical complications, in part because of variability in the presence of linked and unlinked genes that modify the expression of the disease [3, 4].

In Portugal, children with SCA are mainly born in families whose origin is from West Africa (Angola, Cape Verde, São Tomé e Principe and Guiné-Bissau), so the most common haplotypes are Bantu, Benin and Senegal.

Classically clinical different severities were described in different haplotypes (like increased severity in Bantu, and milder in Senegal), with laboratory differences as well (total hemoglobin and HbF levels may be slightly lower in patients with the Bantu haplotype and higher in those with the Senegal one) [5].

Besides S haplotypes, others probably more important factors are the presence of alpha-globin deletions and the Hemoglobin F (HbF) levels since they modify red cell indices and rheology, and positively influence clinical events [6,7]. Absence of co-inheriting alpha-thalassemia and low hemoglobin F levels tend to be associated with more hemolysis, lower hemoglobin oxygen saturations, greater proportions of elevated tricuspid regurgitant jet velocity and brain natriuretic peptide and increased left ventricular mass index [8].

Fetal Hemoglobin is the major modifier of the clinical features of sickle cell anemia and Beta thalassemia. The suggestion that HbF may be responsible for the lack of clinical symptoms in newborns with SCD, was first made by Watson in 1948 [9], who reported that the occurrence of clinical symptoms of SCD started with a decline in HbF levels. Since then, it is now appreciated, that HbF is among the most important known modifiers of the clinical course of SCD. Fetal hemoglobin is believed to decrease hemolysis, and therefore the many complications of SCD, since both fetal hemoglobin ($\alpha_2\gamma_2$) and the mixed hybrid hemoglobin tetramers that it forms ($\alpha_2\gamma\beta^s$) do not participate in the polymerization of the deoxy-sickle hemoglobin [10].

HbF compensates for the deficit of normal Hb A in Beta thalassemia and inhibits deoxygenated sickle hemoglobin (HB S) polymerization, which is the main factor responsible for the vaso-occlusive events and the disease severity (not directly linked to chronic hemolysis and immunodeficiency) [11].

A wide range of HbF expression has been observed among SCD patients from various parts of the world. Many people from the Middle East and India co-inherited additional genetic mutations that allow for the persistence of HbF production, so, as a population, they appear to have less severe disease. Also the several haplotypes of the hemoglobin S gene that correlate with region of origin of the mutation are associated with variation in the expression of HbF: for example within sub-Saharan Africa those with the Bantu haplotype have the lowest HbF expression, while those with the Senegal haplotype the highest [12].

Therapeutic agents that increase HbF expression, such as azacytidine, decitabine, butyrate derivatives, and hydroxyurea, have been investigated in clinical trials to ameliorate the complications of SCD. Hydroxyurea is the only agent yet approved for the prevention of complications of SCD and polymorphisms in the *SAR1A* gene and *TOX* gene may contribute to the variability in HbF response to hydroxyurea.

Early studies have established a level of greater than 10%-20% as a protective cut-off [13].

Efforts persist to identify predictors associated with HbF production in response to hydroxycarbamide: baseline values, white blood cell count and absolute reticulocyte count, but none of these can accurately predict, because the degree of HbF induced by hydroxyurea has a strong heritable component [14].

Genome wide association studies in sickle cell anemia have identified some single nucleotide polymorphism that jointly explain 10-20% variability of HbF, and may be used to predict HbF levels [15].

Being the major modifier of the clinical features of sickle cell anemia, if it were possible to know at birth the HbF level likely to be present after stabilization of this measurement at approximately 5 years of age, a better patient specific prognosis may be given and better tailored treatments could be done. In fact the early prediction of HbF levels might help foresee some complications and guide decisions to pursue HbF induction therapies [11].

Some models have been created to try to predict HbF levels and a Genetic Risk Score (GRS) explains 23.4% of the variability in HbF but does not explain the variability in HbF that is due to heritability estimated in 60-90% [16].

In fact we already know that HbF greater levels are best achieved when treatment is initiated before the natural decline that occurs in children [17].

Another important fact is the presence of alpha-globin deletion. The primary effect of concomitant α-thalassemia is to limit the supply of α globins and thus further favor the competition of non-sickle β globin (γ globin) in the intracellular struggle for available α globins. This lowers the intracellular HbS content and thus prolongs the delay time for HbS polymerization. The resulting erythrocytes are more deformable because they have higher membrane area to volume ration; hence they have less potassium loss and cellular dehydration and a lower mean corpuscular hemoglobin concentration (MCHC). Patients with SCD and α-thalassemia tend to have smaller, lighter cells with a higher circulating Hb concentration and lower rate of hemolysis. Indeed α-thalassemia trait combined with SCD has been associated with a lower risk of cerebral vascular abnormalities and stroke, a finding recently confirmed in a large cohort of children with SCD. However this combination does not necessarily translate into a better clinical outcome, because α-thalassemia has been associated with more vaso-occlusive pain episodes, renal infarction, and avascular necrosis (AVN) of the femoral head. This may be the result of increased hematocrit and concomitant increase in viscosity in certain organs [18].

α-Thalassemia (αα/α- or α-/α-) is present in approximately 1/3 of SCD patients and seems to lessen the clinical severity of disease by decreasing the mean corpuscular hemoglobin concentration, percentage of dense cells, degree of hemolysis and number of irreversibly sickled cells, and by increasing total hemoglobin levels and hemoglobin A2 levels. There seems to be a decreased incidence of involvement of vital organs in SCD patients with alpha-thalassemia and alpha-thalassemia appears to increase survival in certain populations [19].

α-Thalassemia (frequency of one or two α gene deletions is 35% in African-Americans) may be co-inherited with sickle cell trait or disease. Individuals who have both α thalassemia and sickle cell disease (SS) tend to be less anemic than those who have sickle cell disease (SS) alone. The co-inheritance of sickle cell disease and alpha thalassemia trait is associated with a reduction in the risk of some complications, such as stroke, but has no effect on the frequency or severity of vaso-occlusive pain episodes [20].

The effect of alpha-thalassemia is not always beneficial, because some complications such as aseptic necrosis and retinal disease occur more frequently in patients with concurrent alpha-thalassemia [21].

Besides the genetics and all the prediction models mentioned in several studies, environment issues are also important. In this matter sleep is certainly one of them, because sleep is the ultimate human resource to homeostasis.

Sleep in children with SCD have not yet been well characterized in spite of many studies that point a major incidence of sleep disorders [22].

Children and adolescents with Sickle Cell Disease (SCD) usually have a disturbed sleep comparing to controls without SCD.

There is existing evidence that children with SCD are at increased risk of disordered breathing and Obstructive Sleep Apnea (OSA) during sleep. Although the prevalence of sleep disordered breathing is not established in this population estimates range from 5-79% [23] and are far greater than the prevalence of 1-4% in children without SCD [24] partially related with excessive adenoidal and tonsillar growth that occurs, phenomena attributed to compensatory lymphoid tissue hyperplasia or chronic infection secondary to functional asplenia [25].

In children, it is also recognized that adenotonsillar hyperthrophy is the main risk factor for OSA and this results in transient periods of hypoxemia, which may pose a risk for eritrocyte sickling [26].

But it is also known that nearly half of children with SCD, experience nocturnal hypoxemia that is not associated with sleep disordered breathing [27].

In fact there might be other anatomic abnormalities such as those affecting their craniofacial structure particularly due to extramedullary hematopoiesis and/or functional factors that may increase upper airway collapsibility [28].

The disruption of sleep during pain episodes related to vaso-occlusive crisis is an important issue [29] and a better management of pain can improve sleep in these children [30]. In fact pain episodes, not only disrupts sleep but may reduce Stage N3 sleep (Slow Wave Sleep) that has a restorative power and modify pain sensitivity and tolerance [31].

Children with SCD have an increased risk for sleep-disordered breathing and usually they present a lower O_2 saturation than other children with the same severity of obstructive sleep apnea (OSA) but without SCD [32].

Hypoxemia during sleep, increases the risk of vaso-occlusive episodes and acute chest syndrome and is also responsible for a lower degree of executive function, since the time spent with SpO_2 <95% is associated with lower intelligence coefficient (IQ) and with more arousals that can compromise Slow Wave Sleep (SWS) [2].

Nocturnal enuresis is also more frequent in children with SCD and also disruptive of sleep quality (and family quality of life and self esteem) [33].

Ethnicity and low Socioeconomic Status (SES) are also related to poor sleep quality, and these are relevant issues in this population in Portugal, and in general in Europe, being part of recent migrated groups [34].

It is also important to study sleep habits in this population, namely total sleep time, bed time behavior, bed and room conditions, diurnal naps and night waking, as well as parasomnias and excessive day time sleepiness. Also study other sleep variables such as co-sleeping, common in our patients related to cultural issues, and child sleep environment such as shared room, noise, presence of TV should be an interesting investigation.

Parents of children with more severe type of disease, reported more restless sleep, and genotype, was a disease variable that remain significant in regression models suggesting that the severity of disease plays a role in sleep disruption.

Another aspect that should be considered, is the presence of possible allergens or even the diagnosis of asthma, since these children may have a more compromised sleep, exhibiting shorter sleep times, increase night waking and a reduction in N3 sleep stage correlated with asthma severity, and the presence of asthma is associated with an increased risk of pain and acute chest syndrome which may cause a more disturbed sleep [35].

Studying sleep in this population is crucial to understand the relationship between sleep and more serious phenotypes of SCD, and should be included in the regular follow up and orientation of these patients. This fact is related to the knowledge that we need to reduce sleep disturbances that may influence immunity, cognitive development and risk of cardiovascular diseases.

In fact, there are few studies that analyzed polysomnographic characteristics in these children. One of these studies analyzed the polysomnographic data in a sample of 55 children referred for evaluation of sleep disordered breathing, and compared across SCD genotype, age groups and OSA/ adenotonsillectomy conditions, concluding that these children have a unique susceptibility to develop sleep disordered breathing and other sleep related disorders [36].

Considering this point we analyzed polysomnographic sleep characteristics in a sample of children and adolescents with sickle cell disease that were previously studied regarding S haplotype, presence of alpha thalassemia and HbF level.

We conducted a retrospective study that included 54 children and adolescents with SCD.

The population was selected from the Pediatric Sleep Pathology outpatient clinic, in a second level hospital in Amadora-Portugal, where they were sent to evaluate sleep and an eventually sleep disordered breathing following the Sickle Cell Disease Pediatric Group protocol of the Pediatric Department of our Hospital. All patients, aged 1 - 18 years, were previously submitted to a genetic characterization (S haplotype and alpha globin) and Hemoglobin F basal level was determined [37,38]. The level of HbF considered for analysis was the one determined nearer the sleep study evaluation date.

Considering their haplotype, alpha deletion status and HbF level, sleep characteristics were studied.

In pediatric groups, regarding the evidence of obstructive sleep apnea (OSA) and consequently hypoxemia, is notorious an age difference in adenoids and tonsils hypertrophy contribution, so our study group was subdivided in two: a younger group (A, 1-8 years of age) and an older one (B, 9-18 years of age).

A polysomnographic study type 1 (PSG) was performed in all subjects using Alice 5 Respironics®, between July 2010 and June 2013. All PSG were performed using electroencephalogram (frontal, central, and occipital channels) chin electromyogram, two leg channels, electroculogram, piezoelectric chest and abdominal belts, simultaneous pressure transducer and thermistor for nasal flow, transcutaneous (Tc) CO_2 and SpO_2 monitoring, snore microphone, electrocardiogram and simultaneous video monitoring.

All PSG were scored by the same professional, adequately qualified in PSG analysis (Master Sleep Science degree).

Detailed sleep parameters, including total sleep time (TST), wake after sleep onset (WASO), NREM (light and deep slow wave sleep), and REM sleep (rapid eye movements), sleep latency, sleep efficiency, REM and slow wave sleep (SWS) percentage, snoring percentage, Apnea-Hypopnea Index (AHI), and oxygen saturation mean and nadir were considered. Tc CO_2 was not analyzed since values were not available in all individuals. Periodic leg movements and PLM arousal index, enuresis, and parasomnias were also investigated.

The polysomnographic studies were scored considering AASM 2012 rules[39] with the following definitions:

1. Obstructive apnea was defined as the cessation of airflow for two respiratory cycles in presence of continued or increased inspiratory effort throughout the entire period of absent airflow.
2. Hypopnea was defined as a decreased in amplitude of airflow signal >30% of pre-event baseline, lasting two respiratory cycles and accompanied by oxygen desaturation of >3%.
3. An AHI>1/hour was considered diagnostic for OSA Syndrome.
4. Habitual snoring was defined as snoring not accompanied by oxygen desaturation, arousals or changes in airflow.
5. Periodic limb movements of sleep were defined as repetitive jerking of the legs during sleep of more than five movements per hour, 0.5–10 sec in duration, in clusters of four or more separated by 5–90 sec.
6. Arousal defined by an abrupt shift of EEG frequency including alpha, theta and /or frequencies greater than 16Hz (but not spindles) that last at least 3 seconds, with at least 10 seconds of stable sleep preceding the change.
7. Enuresis was defined by recurrent involuntary voiding during sleep at least twice a week in children older than 5 years.
8. Parasomnias were defined by occurrence of confusional arousal, sleepwalking episodes, sleep terrors and nightmare disorders as ICSD-2nd ed [40].

In data analysis, categorical data was expressed as percentage and quantitative data as mean statistic; standard deviation and 95% confidence intervals were also calculated. Differences between groups were calculated by T-Student test. A *p* value of $p \leq 0.05$ was considered significant. All statistic analyses were performed by SPSS statistic software package (SPSS for Windows v22, SPSS Inc, Chicago, IL).

A sample of 54 children and adolescents with SCD was retrospectively studied. Children and adolescents´ age varied from 1 to 18 years, mean 9.52 years; s.d. 4.1 and 55.6% are male.

Regarding adenoid and tonsils hypertrophy, two groups were formed: group A, n= 21, aged 1-8 years (age mean 5.24 years; s.d. 1.78 years, 57.1% male) and group B, n= 33, aged 9-18 years, (age mean 12.24 years; s.d. 2.48 years, 54.5% male).

In the haplotype determination, Bantu/Bantu was predominant, 57.4% of children. The distribution of different haplotypes was Bantu/Bantu n= 31 (group A n= 14; group B n= 17); Senegal/Senegal n=8 (group A n=1; group B n= 7); Bantu/Benin n= 7 (group A n= 4; group B n= 3); Bantu /Senegal n=5 (group A n=0; group B n= 5); atipic Bantu n= 2 (group A n=1; group B n=1); Benin /Benin n= 1 (group A n=1; group B n= 0).

Table 1. Demographic data and haplotype distribution

	Study group (n-54)	**Group A 1-8y (n-21)**	**Group B 9-18y (n-33)**
Mean Age	9.5 y (s.d.±4.1)	5.2 y (s.d.±1.7)	12.2 y (s.d.±2.4)
Gender	55.6% M: 44.4% F	57.1% M:42.9% F	54.5% M:45.5%F
Haplotype (n)			
Bantu/Bantu	31	14	17
Senegal/Senegal	8	1	7
Bantu/Benin	7	4	3
Bantu/Senegal	5	0	5
Atipic Bantu	2	1	1
Benin/Benin	1	1	0

Polysomnographic Results

In this sample, Total Sleep Time (TST) had mean 429.6 minutes (min); s.d. 52.0 (265-516 min).

The shorter TST (265 min) was in a child with Senegal /Senegal haplotype and the longest (516 min) was in a child with the Benin/Benin haplotype. Considering the two groups, TST mean in group A was 444.9 min; s.d. 39.1 and in group B was 419.9 min; s.d. 57.2.

Wake after sleep onset (WASO) had mean 48.4 min; s.d. 42.3 (4.5-200 min). The shorter WASO (4.5 min) was in a child with Bantu/Bantu haplotype and the longest (200 min) was in a child with Senegal/Senegal haplotype. Considering the two groups, in group A, WASO was mean 31.4 min; s.d. 19.8, and in group B, WASO was mean 59.1min; s.d. 49.2.The analysis was statistically significant with $p < 0.02$.

Sleep latency, the duration of time between when lights are turned off as the patient attempts to sleep, until the time patient actually falls asleep, as evidence by EEG and behavioral parameters changes consistent with sleep, was normal in 45 (83.3%) subjects and had mean 20.2 min; s.d. 14.1 (0-67 min) and was longer than 30 min in 10 individuals (5 Bantu/Bantu, 3 Senegal/Senegal, 1 Bantu/Senegal and 1 Bantu/Benin). Considering the two groups, latency mean in group A was 20.7 min; s.d. 14.2 and in group B was mean 20.0 min; s.d. 14.2.

Sleep efficiency, the percentage of total time in bed actually spent in sleep, was normal in 37 (68.5%) subjects and had mean 87.0% (52.3-98.5 %); s.d 9.4. It was shorter than 85% in 17 individuals (6 Bantu/Bantu, 6 Senegal/Senegal, 2 Bantu/Senegal, 1 Bantu/Benin, 1 Benin/Benin and 1 atipic Bantu). Considering the two groups, in group A sleep efficiency had mean 90.4%; s.d. 4.8, and in group B had mean 84.9%; s.d. 11.0. The analysis was statistically significant with $p < 0.04$.

REM latency, the time from sleep onset to the first epoch of REM sleep, was normal in 18 (33.3%) subjects and had mean 155 min (50.5-318 min); s.d. 63.7. It was longer than 120 min in 36 individuals (21 Bantu/Bantu, 6 Senegal/Senegal, 4 Bantu/Senegal,3 Bantu/Benin, 1 Benin/ Benin, and 1 atipic Bantu).Considering the two groups, REM latency mean in group A was 130.3 min; s.d. 54.2, and in group B was 171.6 min; s.d. 64.8. The analysis was statistically significant with $p < 0.02$.

Regarding sleep phases, N1 was normal (0-5%) in 34 subjects and had mean 4.8% (0.1-16.9 %); s.d.3.7. Twenty individuals had N1 phase longer than 5%. From these 9 had Bantu/Bantu, 5 Senegal/Senegal, 3 Bantu/Senegal, 2 Bantu/Benin and 1 atipic Bantu. Considering the two groups, in group A, N1 was mean 3.4%; s.d. 1.9, and in group B, N1 was mean 5.7%; s.d. 4.3. The analysis was statistically significant with $p < 0.03$.

N2 was normal (45-55%) in only 4 subjects: 2 Bantu/Benin, 1 atipic Bantu and 1 Bantu/Bantu, and presented mean 64.9 % (50.2-81,0);s.d. 6.6. Considering the two groups, in group A, N2 was mean 63.2%; s.d. 6.4, and in group B, N2 was mean 66.0%; s.d. 6.7.

N3 had mean 17.5 (1.8-29.9 %); s.d. 6.5 % and was normal (15-20%) in 17 (31.4%) subjects, being shorter than 15% in 16 individuals (9 Bantu/Bantu, 4 Senegal/Senegal, 2 Bantu/Senegal and 1 Bantu/Benin) and longer than 20% in 21 individuals (9 Bantu/Bantu, 5 Bantu/Benin, 3 Senegal/Senegal ,2 Bantu/Senegal, 1 Benin/Benin, and 1 atipic Bantu).Considering the two groups, in group A, N3 was mean 20.2%; s.d. 5.4, and in group B, N3 was mean 15.8%; s.d. 6.7. The analysis was statistically significant with $p <0.02$.

REM was normal (20-25%) in only 3 subjects (1 Senegal/Senegal, 1 Bantu/Benin and 1 Bantu/Bantu) and had mean 12.3 (4.3-21.9%); s.d. 3.9. Considering the two groups, in group A, REM was mean 13.0%; s.d. 3.7, and in group B, REM was mean 11.9%; s.d. 4.1.

Arousals mean was 13.0/h (4.4-28.1); s.d. 4.4 and were above normal (>14/h) in 19 subjects (35.1%) (10 Bantu/Bantu, 5 Senegal/Senegal, 2 Bantu/Senegal, 1 atipic Bantu, 1 Bantu/Benin). In group A mean was 11.3/h; s.d. 3.5 and in group B mean was 14.0/h; s.d.4.6. The analysis was statistically significant with $p <0.02$.

Regarding respiratory events only 4 (7.4%) subjects had a normal AHI (<1/h), 3 Bantu/Bantu and 1 Senegal/Senegal, none submitted to adenotonsillectomy, two had 3 years old and two, 16 years old. Forty-two individuals had light OSA (AHI 1-5/h) (24 Bantu/Bantu, 6 Bantu/Benin, 5 Bantu/Senegal, 5 Senegal/Senegal, 1 atipic Bantu and 1 Benin/Benin) and 8 (14.8%) had moderate OSA (AHI 5 - 10/h) (4 Bantu/Bantu, 2 Senegal/Senegal, 1 atipic Bantu and 1 Bantu/Benin). AHI mean was 3.5/h (0.4-9.5); s.d. 1.7. Considering the two groups, in group A mean was 3.4/h; s.d 1.3 and in group B was 3.5/h; s.d. 1.9.

Mean Sp O_2 was 94.6% (87-99 %); s.d. 3.0, but it was below 90 % in 3 (5.5%) subjects (2 Bantu/Bantu, 1 Bantu/Benin). Considering the two groups in group A mean was 95.2%; s.d. 3.0 and in group B mean was 94.2%; s.d. 3.0.

Minimum Sp O_2 mean was 90.0% (72-97%); s.d. 5.3 and was below 90% in 20 (37%) subjects (10 Bantu/Bantu, 4 Bantu/Benin, 2 Bantu/Senegal, 2 Senegal/Senegal, 1 atipic Bantu and 1 Benin/Benin). Considering the two groups, in group A mean was 89.9%; s.d. 6.6 and in group B mean was 90.0%; s.d. 4.5.

Regarding Periodic Leg Movement (PLM), mean was 3.2/h (0.3-6.3/h); s.d. 1.3 but it was increased (> 5/h) in 6 subjects (11.1%). PLM Arousal Index had mean 2.3/h (0.3-5.1); s.d. 0.9.

Table 2. Sleep and PSG parameters between sub-groups

	Study group 1-18 y (n-54)	**Sub-group A 1-8y (n-21)**	**Sub-group B 9-18y (n-33)**	**p**
TST (min)	429.6 (s.d.±52.0)	444.9 (s.d.±39.1)	419.9 (s.d.±57.2)	0.09
WASO (min)	48.4(s.d.±42.3)	31.4 (s.d.±19.8)	59.1(s.d.±49.2)	**0.02**
Latency (min)	20.3(s.d.±14.1)	20.7 (s.d.±14.3)	20.0(s.d.±14.2)	0.86
Efficiency (%)	87.1 (s.d.±9.4)	90.4 (s.d.±4.8)	84.9 (s.d.±11.0)	**0.04**
REM sleep latency (min)	155.6(s.d.±63.7)	130.3(s.d.±54.2)	171.6(s.d.±64.8)	**0.02**
N1 (%)	4.8 (s.d.±3.7)	3.4 (s.d.±1.9)	5.78 (s.d.±4.3)	**0.03**
N2 (%)	64.9 (s.d.±6.6)	63.2 (s.d.±6.4)	66.0 (s.d.±6.7)	0.14
N3 (%)	17.5 (s.d.±6.5)	20.3 (s.d.±5.4)	15.8 (s.d.±6.7)	**0.02**
REM (%)	12.3 (s.d.±3.9)	13.0 (s.d.±3.7)	11.9 (s.d.±4.1)	0.32
Arousals (n/h)	13,0 (s.d.±4.4)	11.3 (s.d.±3.5)	14.1 (s.d.±4.6)	**0.02**
AHI (n/h)	3.5 (s.d.±1.7)	3.4 (s.d.±1.3)	3.5 (s.d.±1.9)	0.79
Mean SpO2(%)	94.6 (s.d.±3,0)	95.2 (s.d.±3.0)	94.2 (s.d.±3.0)	0.24
Minimum SpO2(%)	90.0 (s.d.±5.3)	89.9 (s.d.±6.6)	90.0 (s.d.±4.5)	0.94
PLM (n/h)	3.2(s.d.±1.3)	3.4 (s.d.±0.9)	2.3 (s.d.±0.6)	0.24
PLM AI (n/h)	2.3(s.d.±0.9)	3.0 (s.d.±1.6)	2.4 (s.d.±1.2)	0.87

In the group, 34 subjects (63%) snored and 37 (68.5%) mentioned disturbed sleep characterized by arousals, excessive movement and sweating.

In this cohort, 8 subjects (14.8%) had a previous adenotonsillectomy, from these 6 had Bantu/Bantu haplotype and 2 had Senegal/Senegal haplotype. One belonged to group A and the other 7 to group B.

Parasomnias were present in 12 individuals, mainly confusional arousal and night terrors in younger children. Sleep walking was not observed.

Nocturnal enuresis was present in 20 (37%) subjects, three still use diapers.

In 39 subjects, VGM was < 80 fL, being assumed that a thalassemia was present. In 23 individuals (42.5%) an alpha deletion was identified, mostly 3.7 deletion. Only one subject had 4.1 deletion. From the total (39) sixteen individuals belonged to group A and 23 to group B. From these, 22 (56.4%) reported snoring and 21 (53.8%) reported disturbed sleep.

Polysomnographic and respiratory parameters were compared between subjects with VGM <80 fL (A< or B <) and those with VGM >80 fL (A> or B>).

Table 3. PSG parameters comparing group A (1-8 years) regarding VGM

	Group A 1-8y (n-21)		
	VGM<80 (A<) (n-16)	**VGM>80 (A>) (n-5)**	**p**
TST (min)	438.1 (s.d.±37.1)	466.4 (s.d.±41.4)	0.17
WASO (min)	25.7(s.d.±10.9)	49.7(s.d.±31.2)	**0.01**
Latency (min)	21.2 (s.d.±16.0)	19.1 (s.d.±7.3)	0.78
Efficiency (%)	87.9 (s.d.±5.9)	91.3 (s.d.±4.2)	0.17
REM sleep latency (min)	125.5 (s.d.±41.2)	145.7 (s.d.±89.0)	0.48
N1 (%)	3.2 (s.d.±2.0)	4.0 (s.d.±1.7)	0.44
N2 (%)	63.3 (s.d.±6.5)	62.9 (s.d.±6.9)	0.89
N3 (%)	20.5 (s.d.±5.6)	19.2 (s.d.±5.0)	0.65
REM (%)	12.8 (s.d.±3.1)	13.7 (s.d.±5.6)	0.66
Arousals (n/h)	11.0 (s.d.±2.7)	12.0 (s.d.±5.7)	0.59
AHI (n/h)	3.3 (s.d.±1.4)	3.6 (s.d.±1.1)	0.71
Mean SpO_2 (%)	95.5 (s.d.±3.1)	94.4 (s.d.±2.7)	0.47
Minimum SpO_2 (%)	91.0 (s.d.±5.4)	85.7 (s.d.±10.0)	0.16

In group A (younger children), A< n= 16 and A> n=5, this analysis was statistically significant regarding WASO with p value < 0.01.

Regarding polysomnographic parameters: TST was mean 438.1 min; s.d. 37.1 in A< and 466.4 min; s.d. 41.4 in A >; WASO was mean 25.7 min; s.d. 10.9 in A< and 49.7 min; s.d. 31.2 in A>; Latency was mean 21.2 min; s.d. 16.0 in A< and 19.1 min; s.d. 7.3 in A>; REM latency was mean 125.5 min; s.d. 41.2 in A< and 145.7 min; s.d. 89.0 in A>. Efficiency was mean 87.9 %; s.d. 5.9 in A< and 91.3%; s.d.4.2 in A>;N1 was mean 3.2%; s.d. 2.0 in A< and 4.0%; s.d. 1.7 in A>; N2 was mean 63.3 %; s.d. 6.5 in A< and 62.9 %; s.d. 6.9

in A>; N3 was mean 20.5%;s.d. 5.6 in A< and 19.2%; s.d. 5.0 in A>; REM was mean 12.8%; s.d. 3.1 in A< and 13.7%; s.d. 5.6 in A>; Arousals were mean 11.0/h; s.d. 2.7 in A< and 12.0/h; s.d. 5.7 in A>.

Regarding respiratory parameters, AHI was mean 3.3/h; s.d. 1.4 in A< and 3.6/h; s.d. 1.1 in A>. Mean Sp O_2 was 95.5%; s.d.3.1 in A< and 94.4%; s.d. 2.7 in A>.Minimum Sp O_2 was mean 91.0%; s.d. 5.4 in A< and 85.7%; s.d. 10.0 in A >.

In group B, older children and adolescents, the VGM was determined in only 23 subjects. Fourteen had VGM <80fL (B<), and 9 had VGM >80fL (B>). This analysis was statistically significant regarding N1 with a p value < 0.00.

Regarding polysomnographic parameters: TST was mean 434,6 min;s.d. 43.2 in B< and 426.5 min;s.d.52.0 in B >; WASO was mean 39.7 min; s.d. 27.1 in B< and 66.2 min; s.d. 50.6 in B>; Latency was mean 20.9 min; s.d. 16.2 in B< and 15.7 min; s.d. 13.0 in B>;REM latency was mean 162.6 min; s.d. 59.7 in B< and 165.3 min; s.d. 69.2 in B>; Efficiency was mean 88.8 %; s.d. 7.3 in B< and 84.0%; s.d. 10.2 in B>; N1 was mean 3.6%; s.d. 2.6 in B< and 7.8%; s.d. 3.8 in B>; N2 was mean 69.2 %; s.d. 6.1 in B< and 66.9 %; s.d. 6.1 in B>; N3 was mean 14.1 %;s.d. 5.5 in B< and 14.6 %; s.d. 7.8 in B>; REM was mean 12.0%; s.d. 3.1 in B< and 10.5%; s.d. 3.0 in B>; Arousals were mean 14.2/h; s.d. 3.7 in B< and 12.3/h; s.d. 3.2 in B>;

Regarding respiratory parameters, AHI was mean 3.4/h; s.d. 1.4 in B< and 3.4/h; s.d. 1.6 in B>;Mean Sp O_2 was 95.0%; s.d.2.4 in B< and 93.1%; s.d. 3.1 in B>; Minimum Sp O_2 was mean 91.4%; s.d. 2.6 in B< and 90.0%; s.d. 4.0 in B >.

Comparing the two groups of subjects, A (n=16) younger and B (n=14) older, with VGM < 80fL, this analysis was statistically significant regarding REM sleep latency ($p < 0.05$), N2 ($p<0.01$), N3 ($p<0.00$) and number of arousals ($p<0.01$)

Regarding polysomnographic parameters: TST was mean 438,1 min;s.d. 37.1 in A and 434.6 min;s.d.43.2 in B; WASO was mean 25.7 min; s.d. 10.9 in A and 39.7 min; s.d. 27.1 in B; Latency was mean 21.2min; s.d. 16.0 in A and 20.9 min; s.d. 16.2 in B; REM latency was mean 125.5 min; s.d. 41.2 in A and 162.6 min; s.d. 59.7 in B; Efficiency was mean 91.2%; s.d. 4.2 in A and 88.8%; s.d. 7.3 in B; N1 was mean 3.2%; s.d. 2.0 in A and 3.6%; s.d. 2.6 in B; N2 was mean 63.3 %; s.d. 6.5 in A and 69.2 %; s.d. 6.1 in B; N3 was mean 20.5 %;s.d. 5.6 in A and 14.1 %; s.d. 5.5 in B; REM was mean 12.8%; s.d. 3.1 in A and 12.0%; s.d. 3.1 in B; Arousals were mean 11.0/h; s.d. 2.7 in A and 14.2/h; s.d. 3.7 in B.

Table 4. PSG parameters comparing group B (9-18 years) regarding VGM

	Group B 9-18y (n-23)		
	VGM<80 (B<) (n-14)	VGM>80 (B>) (n-9)	p
TST (min)	434.6 (s.d.±43.2)	426.5 (s.d.±52.0)	0.69
WASO (min)	39.7(s.d.±27.1)	66.2 (s.d.±50.6)	0.12
Latency (min)	20.9 (s.d.±16.2)	15.7 (s.d.±13.0)	0.43
Efficiency (%)	88.8 (s.d.±7.3)	84.0 (s.d.±10.2)	0.20
REM sleep latency (min)	162.6 (s.d.±59.7)	165.3 (s.d.±69.2)	0.92
N1 (%)	3.6 (s.d.±2.6)	7.8 (s.d.±3.8)	**0.00**
N2 (%)	69.2 (s.d.±6.1)	66.9 (s.d.±6.1)	0.40
N3 (%)	14.1 (s.d.±5.5)	14.6 (s.d.±7.8)	0.87
REM(%)	12.0 (s.d.±3.1)	10.5 (s.d.±3.0)	0.26
Arousals (n/h)	14.2 (s.d.±3.7)	12.3 (s.d.±3.2)	0.23
AHI (n/h)	3.4(s.d.±1.4)	3.4 (s.d.±1.6)	0.92
Mean SpO_2(%)	95.0 (s.d.±2.4)	93.1 (s.d.±3.1)	0.11
Minimum SpO_2(%)	91.4 (s.d.±2.6)	90.0 (s.d.±4.0)	0.32

Regarding respiratory parameters: AHI was mean 3.3/h; s.d. 1.4 in A and 3.4/h; s.d. 1.4 in B; Mean Sp O_2 was 95.5%; s.d.3.1 in A and 95.0%; s.d. 2.4 in B; Minimum Sp O_2 was mean 91.0%; s.d. 5.4 in A and 91.4 %; s.d. 2.6 in B.

Comparing the two groups of subjects, A (n=5) younger and B (n=9) older, with VGM > 80fL, the analysis was not statistically significant.

Regarding polysomnographic parameters: TST was mean 466,4 min;s.d. 41.4 in A and 426.5 min;s.d.52.0 in B; WASO was mean 49.7 min; s.d. 31.2 in A and 66.2 min; s.d. 50.6 in B; Latency was mean 19.1min; s.d. 7.3 in A and 15.7 min; s.d. 13.0 in B; REM latency was mean 145.7 min; s.d. 89.0 in A and 165.3 min; s.d. 69.2 in B; Efficiency was mean 87.8%; s.d. 5.9 in A and 84.0%; s.d. 10.2 in B; N1 was mean 4.0%; s.d. 1.7 in A and 7.8 %; s.d. 3.8 in B; N2 was mean 62.9 %; s.d. 6.9 in A and 66.9 %; s.d. 6.1 in B; N3 was mean 19.2 %;s.d. 5.0 in A and 14.6 %; s.d. 7.8 in B; REM was mean 13.7 %; s.d. 5.6 in A and 10.5 %; s.d. 3.0 in B; Arousals were mean 12.0/h; s.d. 5.7 in A and 12.3/h; s.d. 3.2 in B.

Regarding respiratory parameters: AHI was mean 3.6/h; s.d. 1.7 in A and 3.4/h; s.d. 1.6 in B; Mean Sp O_2 was 94.4%; s.d.2.7 in A and 93.1 %; s.d. 3.1 in B; Minimum Sp O_2 was mean 85.7 %; s.d. 10.0 in A and 90.0 %; s.d. 4.0 in B.

Table 5. PSG parameters comparing both groups (A 1-8 years and B 9-18 years) with VGM<80fL

	VGM<80 fL		
	Group A 1-8y (n-16)	**Group B 9-18y (n-14)**	**p**
TST (min)	438.1 (s.d.±37.1)	434.6 (s.d.±43.2)	0.81
WASO(min)	25.7 (s.d.±10.9)	39.7 (s.d.±27.1)	0.07
Latency (min)	21.2 (s.d.±16.0)	20.9 (s.d.±16.2)	0.96
Efficiency (%)	91.2 (s.d.±4.2)	88.8 (s.d.±7.3)	0.27
REM sleep latency (min)	125.5 (s.d.±41.2)	162.6 (s.d.±59.7)	**0.05**
N1 (%)	3.2(s.d.±2.0)	3.6 (s.d.±2.6)	0.67
N2 (%)	63.3 (s.d.±6.5)	69.2 (s.d.±6.1)	**0.01**
N3 (%)	20.5 (s.d.±5.6)	14.1 (s.d.±5.5)	**0.00**
REM(%)	12.8 (s.d.±3.1)	12.1 (s.d.±3.1)	0.52
Arousals (n/h)	11.0 (s.d.±2.7)	14.2 (s.d.±3.7)	**0.01**
AHI (n/h)	3.3 (s.d.±1.4)	3.4 (s.d.±1.4)	0.83
Mean SpO_2(%)	95.5 (s.d.±3.1)	95.0 (s.d.±2.4)	0.64
Minimum SpO_2(%)	91.0 (s.d.±5.4)	91.4 (s.d.±2.6)	0.79

Table 6. PSG parameters comparing both groups (A 1-8 years and B 9-18 years) with VGM>80fL

	VGM>80 fL		
	Group A 1-8y (n-5)	**Group B 9-18y (n-9)**	**p**
TST (min)	466.4 (s.d.±41.4)	426.5 (s.d.±52.0)	0.17
WASO(min)	49.7 (s.d.±31.2)	66.2 (s.d.±50.6)	0.52
Latency (min)	19.1 (s.d.±7.3)	15.7 (s.d.±13.0)	0.61
Efficiency (%)	87.8 (s.d.±5.9)	84.0 (s.d.±10.2)	0.46
REM sleep latency (min)	145.7 (s.d.±89.0)	165.3 (s.d.±69.2)	0.65
N1 (%)	4.0 (s.d.±1.7)	7.8 (s.d.±3.8)	0.07
N2 (%)	62.9 (s.d.±6.9)	66.9 (s.d.±6.1)	0.28
N3 (%)	19.2 (s.d.±5.0)	14.6 (s.d.±7.8)	0.26
REM(%)	13.7 (s.d.±5.6)	10.5 (s.d.±3.0)	0.19
Arousals (n/h)	12.0 (s.d.±5.7)	12.3 (s.d.±3.2)	0.92
AHI (n/h)	3.6 (s.d.±1.7)	3.4 (s.d.±1.6)	0.79
Mean SpO_2(%)	94.4 (s.d.±2.7)	93.1 (s.d.±3.1)	0.46
Minimum SpO_2(%)	85.7 (s.d.±10.0)	90.0 (s.d.±4.0)	0.28

Regarding HbF level when PSG was done, 21 subjects (38.9%) had HbF >10%, 12 from group A and 9 from group B.

When we consider this group with HbF above 10%, and the two age groups, A (1-8 years) and B (9-18 years), analysis was statistically significant regarding TST ($p<0.03$), WASO ($p<0.01$), efficiency ($p<0.00$), N1 ($p<0.05$), N3 ($p<0.05$) and number of arousals ($p<0.04$).

Table 7. PSG parameters comparing both groups (A 1-8 years and B 9-18 years) with Hb F >10%

	HbF>10%		
	Group A 1-8y (n-12)	**Group B 9-18y (n-9)**	**p**
TST (min)	454.5 (s.d.±42.2)	394.3 (s.d.±70.5)	**0.03**
WASO (min)	37.8 (s.d.±22.8)	96.2 (s.d.±59.4)	**0.01**
Latency (min)	24.8 (s.d.±15.3)	26.1 (s.d.±12.7)	0.84
Efficiency (%)	88.9 (s.d.±4.9)	75.8 (s.d.±12.7)	**0.00**
REM sleep latency (min)	134.7 (s.d.±61.2)	174.2(s.d.±75.9)	0.20
N1 (%)	3.7 (s.d.±1.7)	6.6 (s.d.±4.6)	**0.05**
N2 (%)	60.9 (s.d.±6.3)	65.0 (s.d.±4.6)	0.12
N3 (%)	21.9 (s.d.±5.1)	17.4 (s.d.±4.8)	**0.05**
REM (%)	13.4 (s.d.±4.0)	10.8 (s.d.±4.8)	0.21
Arousals (n/h)	11.1(s.d.±4.5)	15.8 (s.d.±5.6)	**0.04**
AHI (n/h)	3.4 (s.d.±1.4)	2.3 (s.d.±1.3)	0.10
Mean SpO_2(%)	96.0 (s.d.±2.2)	95.7 (s.d.±1.6)	0.80
Minimum SpO_2(%)	90.0 (s.d.±7.0)	92.4 (s.d.±3.3)	0.35

Regarding polysomnographic parameters: TST in group A mean was 454.5min; s.d. 42.2 and in group B mean was 394.3 min; s.d. 70.5. Considering WASO, in group A mean was 37.8min; s.d. 22.8, and in group B mean was 96.2 min; s.d. 59.4. Regarding sleep latency, in group A mean was 24.8 min; s.d. 15.3 and in group B mean was 26.1 min; s.d.12.7; REM latency, in group A mean was 134.7 min; s.d. 61.2 and in group B mean was 174.2 min; s.d.75.9; Considering sleep efficiency, in group A, mean was 88.9%; s.d. 4.9, and in group B mean was 75.8%; s.d.12.7; Regarding sleep phases, in N1, in group A, mean was 3.7 %; s.d. 1.7, and in group B mean was 6.6%; s.d.4.6; N2 in group A mean was 60.9%; s.d.6.3 and in group B mean was 65.0%;s.d. 4.6; N3 in group A mean was 21.9%; s.d.5.1 and in group B mean was 17.4%; s.d. 4.8; REM in group A mean was 13.4%; s.d.4.0 and in group B mean was

10.8%;s.d. 4.8; Regarding arousals, in group A, mean was 11.1/h;s.d.4.5 and in group B mean was 15.8/h; s.d. 5.6;

Regarding respiratory parameters: AHI mean was 3.4/h;s.d.1.4 in group A and 2.3/h; s.d. 1.3 in group B. Mean Sp O_2 was 96,0%;s.d. 2.2 in group A and 95.7%; s.d.1.6 in group B. Minimum Sp O_2 mean was 90.0%;s.d. 7.0 in group A and 92.4%; s.d.3.3 in group B.

Considering Hb F lower than 10%, n= 33 (61.1%), in group A n=9 and group B n= 24 the analysis was statistically significant regarding REM sleep latency ($p<0.05$).

Regarding polysomnographic parameters: TST in group A mean was 432,0 min; s.d. 32.3 and in group B mean was 429,5 min; s.d. 49.7; Regarding WASO, in group A mean was 22.8 min,; s.d. 11.3, and in group B mean was 45.2 min; s.d. 37.3; regarding Sleep latency, in group A mean was 15.2 min; s.d. 11.3, and in group B mean was 17.7 min;s.d.14.2; considering REM latency, in group A mean was 124.5 min; s.d. 46.1 and in group B mean was 170.6 min; s.d.61.9; Sleep efficiency, in group A, mean was 92.5 %; s.d. 4.0, and in group B mean was 88.3%; s.d.8.2;Regarding sleep phases, in N1 in group A, mean was 3.1 %; s.d. 2.2, and in group B mean was 5.4%;s.d.4.2; N2 in group A mean was 66.3%; s.d.5.4 and in group B mean was 66.3%; s.d. 7.3; N3 in group A mean was 18.0%; s.d.5.3 and group B mean was 15.3%; s.d. 7.3; REM in group A mean was 12.5%; s.d.3.4 and in group B mean was 12.2%; s.d. 3.8; Regarding arousals, in group A mean was 11.5/h; s.d.1.8 and in group B mean was 13.4/h; s.d. 4.1.

Regarding respiratory parameters and HbF below 10% and considering the two groups, AHI mean was 3.4/h;s.d.1.2 in group A and 4.0/h; s.d. 1.9 in group B. Mean Sp O_2 was 94.3%; s.d. 3.8 in group A and 93.7%; s.d.3.2 in group B. Minimum Sp O_2 mean was 89.8%;s.d. 6.5 in group A and 89.1 %; s.d.4.6 in group B.

Out of all the patients, 30 are medicated with hydroxycarbamide. In group A, from the 13 individuals medicated, 6 had HbF > 10% and 7 had HbF <10%. In group B, 17 are medicated, 14 had HbF > 10% and 3 had HbF <10%.

When comparing subjects that snored with HbF value, from the 34 individuals that mentioned snoring 22 (66.6%) had HbF below 10. Regarding disturbed sleep 22 (66.6%) subjects that mentioned it, had HbF below 10.

From the 8 subjects submitted to adenotonsillectomy, 6 had HbF below 10%.

When comparing the two groups regarding HbF level (< 10% and > 10%) in group A, n=21, younger children, this analysis was statistically significant regarding N2 ($p<0.05$).

Table 8. PSG parameters comparing both groups (A 1-8 years and B 9-18 years) with Hb F <10%

	HbF<10%		
	Group A 1-8y (n-9)	**Group B 9-18y (n-24)**	**p**
TST (min)	432.0 (s.d.±32.3)	429.5 (s.d.±49.7)	0.89
WASO (min)	22.8 (s.d.±11.3)	45.2 (s.d.±37.3)	0.09
Latency (min)	15.2 (s.d.±11.3)	17.7 (s.d.±14.2)	0.65
Efficiency (%)	92.5 (s.d.±4.0)	88.3 (s.d.±8.2)	0.16
REM sleep latency (min)	124.5 (s.d.±46.1)	170.6 (s.d.±61.9)	**0.05**
N1 (%)	3.1 (s.d.±2.2)	5.4 (s.d.±4.2)	0.13
N2 (%)	66.3 (s.d.±5.4)	66.3 (s.d.±7.3)	1.00
N3 (%)	18.0 (s.d.±5.3)	15.3 (s.d.±7.3)	0.33
REM (%)	12.5 (s.d.±3.4)	12.2 (s.d.±3.8)	0.88
Arousals (n/h)	11.5 (s.d.±1.8)	13.4 (s.d.±4.1)	0.19
AHI (n/h)	3.4 (s.d.±1.2)	4.0 (s.d.±1.9)	0.43
Mean SpO_2(%)	94.3 (s.d.±3.8)	93.7 (s.d.±3.2)	0.64
Minimum SpO_2(%)	89.8 (s.d.±6.5)	89.1 (s.d.±4.6)	0.72

Considering polysomnographic parameters: TST and HbF < 10% mean was 432.1 min; s.d.32.3, and with HbF > 10% mean was 454.5 min; s.d.42.2;regarding WASO and HbF < 10% mean was 22.8 min; s.d. 11.3, and with HbF > 10% mean was 37.8 min; s.d.22.8; considering sleep latency and HbF < 10% mean was 15.2 min; s.d. 11.3, and with HbF > 10% mean was 24.8; min s.d.15.3; Considering REM latency and Hb F < 10% mean was 124.5 min; s.d. 46.1, and with HbF >10% mean was 134.7 min s.d.61.2; regarding Sleep efficiency and HbF <10% mean was 92.5%; s.d.4.0 and with HbF > 10% mean was 88.9%; s.d.4.9.Considering sleep phases, in N1 and HbF <10% mean was 3.1%; s.d.2.2 and with HbF > 10%, mean was 3.7%; s.d.1.7; N2 and HbF <10% mean was 66.3%; s.d.5.4 and with HbF > 10%, mean was 60.9%; s.d.6.3; N3 and HbF <10% mean was 18.0%; s.d.5.3 and with HbF > 10%, mean was 21.9%; s.d.5.1; in REM and HbF <10% mean was 12.5%; s.d. 3.4 and with HbF > 10% mean was 13.4%; s.d.4.0.Regarding arousals, HbF <10% mean was 11.5/h; s.d.1.8 and HbF > 10% mean was 11.1/h; s.d.4.5.

Regarding respiratory events, AHI and Hb F <10% mean was 3.4/h; s.d.1.2 and with HbF > 10% mean was 3.4/h; s.d.1.4.Mean Sp O_2 and Hb F <10% was 94.3%; s.d.3.8 and with HbF > 10% mean was 96.0%; s.d.2.2.

Minimum Sp O_2 and Hb F <10% mean was 89.8%; s.d.6.5 and with HbF > 10% mean was 90.0%; s.d.7.0.

Table 9. PSG parameters comparing Hb F level in younger children (group A)

	Group A 1-8y (n-21)		
	HbF<10% (n-9)	**HbF>10% (n-12)**	**p**
TST (min)	432.1 (s.d.±32.3)	454.5 (s.d.±42.2)	0.20
WASO(min)	22.8 (s.d.±11.3)	37.8 (s.d.±22.8)	0.09
Latency (min)	15.2 (s.d.±11.3)	24.8 (s.d.±15.3)	0.13
Efficiency (%)	92.5 (s.d.±4.0)	88.9 (s.d.±4.9)	0.09
REM sleep latency (min)	124.5 (s.d.±46.1)	134.7 (s.d.±61.2)	0.68
N1 (%)	3.1 (s.d.±2.2)	3.7 (s.d.±1.7)	0.51
N2 (%)	66.3 (s.d.±5.4)	60.9 (s.d.±6.3)	**0.05**
N3 (%)	18.0 (s.d.±5.3)	21.9 (s.d.±5.1)	0.10
REM(%)	12.5 (s.d.±3.4)	13.4 (s.d.±4.0)	0.59
Arousals (n/h)	11.5 (s.d.±1.8)	11.1 (s.d.±4.5)	0.83
AHI (n/h)	3.4 (s.d.±1.2)	3.4 (s.d.±1.4)	0.94
Mean SpO_2(%)	94.3 (s.d.±3.8)	96.0 (s.d.±2.2)	0.22
Minimum SpO_2(%)	89.8 (s.d.±6.5)	90.0 (s.d.±7.0)	0.97

When we compare the two groups regarding HbF level (< 10% and > 10%) in group B, n=33, older children and adolescents, this analysis was statistically significant regarding WASO ($p<0.01$), efficiency ($p<0.00$) and AHI ($p<0.03$).

Considering polysomnographic parameters: TST and HbF < 10% mean was 429.5 min; s.d.49.7, and with HbF >10% mean was 394.3 min; s.d.70.5;regarding WASO and HbF < 10% mean was 45.2 min; s.d. 37.3, and with HbF > 10% mean was 96.2 min; s.d.59.4;Considering Sleep latency and Hb F < 10% mean was 17.7 min; s.d. 14.2, and with HbF > 10% mean was 26.1min; s.d.12.7;In REM latency and HbF < 10% mean was 170.6 min; s.d. 61.9, and with HbF > 10% mean was 174.2 min; s.d.75.9; Regarding Sleep efficiency and HbF <10% mean was 88.3; s.d.8.2 and HbF > 10% mean was 75.8%; s.d.12.7; in N1 and HbF <10% mean was 5.4%; s.d.4.2 and with HbF > 10% mean was 6.6%; s.d.4.6; N2 and HbF <10% mean was 66.3%; s.d.7.3 and with HbF > 10% mean was 65.0%; s.d.4.6; N3 and HbF <10% mean was 15.3%; s.d.7.3 and with HbF > 10% mean was 17.4%; s.d.4.8; REM and HbF

<10% mean was 12.2%; s.d. 3.8 and with HbF > 10% mean was 10.8%; s.d.4.8.Regarding arousals and HbF <10% mean was 13.4/h; s.d.4.1 and with HbF > 10% mean was 15.8/h; s.d.5.6.

Regarding respiratory events: AHI and Hb F <10% mean was 4.0/h; s.d.1.9 and with HbF > 10% mean was 2.3/h; s.d.1.3; Mean Sp O_2 and HbF <10% mean was 93.7%; s.d.3.2 and with HbF > 10% mean was 95.7%; s.d.1.6; Minimum Sp O_2 and HbF <10% mean was 89.1%; s.d.4.6 and with HbF >10% mean was 92.4%;s.d.3.3.

Table 10. PSG parameters comparing Hb F level in older children (group B)

	Group B 9-18y (n-33)		
	HbF<10% (n-24)	**HbF>10% (n-9)**	**p**
TST (min)	429.5 (s.d.±49.7)	394.3 (s.d.±70.5)	0.12
WASO(min)	45.2 (s.d.±37.3)	96.2 (s.d.±59.4)	**0.01**
Latency (min)	17.7 (s.d.±14.2)	26.1 (s.d.±12.7)	0.13
Efficiency (%)	88.3 (s.d.±8.2)	75.8 (s.d.±12.7)	**0.00**
REM sleep latency (min)	170.6(s.d.±61.9)	174.2 (s.d.±75.9)	0.89
N1 (%)	5.4 (s.d.±4.2)	6.6 (s.d.±4.6)	0.49
N2 (%)	66.3 (s.d.±7.3)	65.0(s.d.±4.6)	0.62
N3 (%)	15.3 (s.d.±7,3)	17.4 (s.d.±4,8)	0.44
REM (%)	12,2(s.d.±3.8)	10.8 (s.d.±4.8)	0.38
Arousals (n/h)	13.4 (s.d.±4.1)	15.8 (s.d.±5.6)	0.18
AHI (n/h)	4.0 (s.d.±1.9)	2.3 (s.d.±1.3)	**0.03**
Mean SpO_2(%)	93.7 (s.d.±3.2)	95.7 (s.d.±1.6)	0.08
Minimum SpO_2(%)	89.1 (s.d.±4.6)	92.4 (s.d.±3.3)	0.07

To our knowledge this is the first study that analyzes sleep disturbance considering different haplotypes, presence of alpha thalassemia and HbF values.

In children with SCD, when compared to controls [22], sleep is usually shorter and more disturbed, but the analysis in different haplotypes was not found.

It is known that the studied haplotypes have a different severity in the outcome and co morbidities, namely Bantu/Bantu haplotype is considered to have a more severe outcome [5]. But in our study, the most disturbed group was Senegal/Senegal. In fact, the shorter TST was in a child with

Senegal/Senegal haplotype, and the longest with Benin/Benin haplotype which has been referred as least severe of those that were studied. Regarding WASO the longest was also in a child with Senegal/Senegal haplotype. It is evident that sleep disturbances are present in this group of children and regarding sleep efficiency, disturbed in 17 children, 6 of them were Senegal/Senegal; regarding sleep latency from the 10 children that was longer than normal, 3 of them were from Senegal/Senegal haplotype and in REM latency from the 36 children that was longer than normal, 6 of them were from Senegal/Senegal haplotype. Regarding sleep phases, N1 was longer in five children Senegal/Senegal and N3 was diminished in four and longer in three children from this haplotype. Not being statistically significant, related to sample size and distribution of haplotypes, although Bantu/Bantu is considered to be a more severe haplotype, and Senegal/Senegal a less severe one, it seems to be more severe to have Senegal/Senegal haplotype regarding sleep (longer latency, longer WASO, less efficiency and longer N1 so less TST) in spite of many sleep disturbances also found in Bantu/Bantu haplotype. Polysomnographic parameters were similar in all the haplotypes, finding no relevance in HbF level or thalassemic status. It should be interesting to have a larger sample to confirm the collected data.

Considering the two groups of children (A younger and B older) group B had more sleep disturbances: WASO was longer ($p<0.02$) sleep efficiency was shorter ($p<0.04$) and REM latency was longer ($p<0.02$). Regarding sleep phases, N1 was longer ($p<0.03$) and N3 was shorter ($p< 0.02$). Arousals were more significant in group B ($p<0.02$). This fact evidences the more disturbed sleep in older children and adolescents with SCD perhaps related to more co-morbidities and longer evolution especially cardio-vascular and pulmonary.

When considering the presence of microcytosis, this has no significant influence on sleep characteristics. In group A, WASO is longer in A> (VGM > 80Fl) ($p<0.01$) and in group B, N1 was longer in B> ($p<0.00$).When comparing sleep in group A and group B regarding microcytosis (VGM<80fL), REM latency was longer in B ($p<0.05$), N2 was longer in B ($p<0.01$), N3 was shorter in group B ($p<0.00$) and arousals was more frequent in B ($p<0.01$) which means that, in older children, in spite of a considered protective factor given by microcytosis [19] there is a more disturbed sleep with a phase N2 of slow wave sleep being more prolonged which is deleterious, and a shorter phase N3, since we know that deep slow wave sleep (N3) has a more restorative role regarding sleep functions. This fact may also be explained by the small sample that we studied. When we analyzed the two groups without microcytosis no statistical difference was found meaning that sleep parameters were similar.

Considering HbF level, that is admitted to be protective [10,12,13] it is interesting to notice that, when we compare HbF < 10% in the 2 groups (A and B), REM latency is longer in group B ($p<0.05$) which has importance regarding potential biological markers. This fact is considered to be related with REM suppression medications such as barbiturates and tricyclic anti - depressants and alcohol, but also with sleep apnea, and in fact, in this comparison in group B, AHI is higher, 4.0/h, although not statistically significant [41].

Considering HbF > 10%, which may give some protection regarding more severe disease, the group B, older children, has short TST ($p<0.03$), longer WASO ($p<0.01$) and shorter efficiency ($p< 0.00$). Regarding sleep phases children from group B have longer N1 ($p<0.05$) and shorter N3 ($p<0.05$). Considering arousals, it is more frequent in older children ($p<0.04$). So it shows that, in spite of the protection given by HbF level, older children have more sleep disturbances with less restorative sleep characterized by shorter, more fragmented and lighter sleep.

But when comparing separately each group of children and the level of HbF, in group A, phase N2 is longer when HbF <10% ($p<0.05$) which means that younger children without the protection of HbF, have a lighter sleep that might influence cognitive development. In group B, curiously WASO is longer with HbF > 10% ($p<0.01$) and efficiency is shorter ($p<0.00$). This means that HbF gives no protection regarding sleep duration.

Also when considering sleep respiratory parameters it was found that HbF > 10% in the group of older children gives a statistically significant protection ($p<0.03$) since in this group, children have a lower AHI of 2.3/h, compared with the HbF <10% that have an AHI 4.0/h. This is a very important fact, since it is known that children with SCD have an increased risk of OSA and higher levels of HbF could give them some protection regarding respiratory events. Regarding mean SpO_2 and minimum SpO_2, *p* value is not statistically significant, but in fact with HbF > 10% values are higher so a benefit might exist and in larger sample it might be more evident.

So, in our point of view it might be assumed that HbF could have an important role related to sleep respiratory disturbances, with less hypoxemia during sleep, fact that is a benefit for the occurrence of vaso-occlusive and pain episodes, and highlights the importance of keeping HbF in highest possible levels.

We consider that this study has some limitations namely sample size and age heterogeneity. In literature, the level of HbF as a prognosis value at 5 years of age and we did not take it into consideration, but instead the level of HbF at the time of PSG, fact that can incur on some bias. Also the duration of therapy with hydroxyurea and consequently its influence in the HbF level was not evaluated.

Conclusion

In the last years, family and empirical medical knowledge that sleep is disturbed in children with SCD compared to controls, has been demonstrated and detailed in scientific studies. In this small cohort S haplotype and microcytosis did not seem to significantly influence sleep characteristics (even if Senegal/Senegal haplotype individuals presented more serious sleep disturbances, they had no statistics significance). But the presence of higher levels of HbF seems to be protective regarding respiratory sleep disturbances, mainly AHI, in older children and adolescents with less adenoid and tonsils hypertrophy. This is an important issue that supports the need of pursuing higher levels of HbF in order to benefit sleep and consequently have less sleep disordered breathing, better pain control, less pulmonary and cardiovascular diseases, better school performance and a longer life for these children with SCD. We hope that growing interest in sleep studies in this multi systemic and complex disease helps to develop strategies to improve the patient's quality of life in present and future times.

References

[1] http://www.who.int/genomics/public/Maphaemoglobin.pdf, last accessed at March, 13 2015.

[2] Hollocks, M; Kok, T; Kirkham, F; Gavlak, J; Inusa, B; De Baun, M; Haan, M. Nocturnal Oxygen desaturation and disordered sleep as a Potential factor in executive dysfunction in Sickle Cell Anemia. J Int Neuropsychol Soc., 2012 Jan, 18(10), 168-173.

[3] A., Driss; K.O., Asare; J.M., Hibbert; B.E., Gee; T.V. Adamkiewicz, J.K. Stiles. Sickle Cell Disease in the Post Genomic Era: A

Monogenic Disease with a Polygenic Phenotype, Genomics Insights., 2009 July 30, 2009(2), 23–48.

[4] Martins, R; Morais, A; Dias, A; Soares, I; Rolão, C; Ducla-Soares, JL, et al. Early modification of sickle cell disease clinical course by UDP-glucuronosyltransferase 1A1 gene promoter polymorphism. J Hum Genet., 2008, 53(6), 524-8. doi: 10.1007/s10038-008-0281-3.

[5] Nagel, RL; Fabry, ME; Pagnier, J; Zohoun, I; Wajcman, H; Baudin, V; Labie, D. Hematologically and genetically distinct forms of sickle cell anemia in Africa. The Senegal type and the Benin type. N Engl J Med., 1985 Apr 4, 312(14), 880-4.

[6] Van, Enk, A; Lang, A; White, JM; Lehmann, H. Benign obstetric history in women with sickle-cell anaemia associated with -thalassaemia..Br Med J., 1972 Dec 2, 4(5839), 524-6.

[7] Sankaran, VG; Lettre, G; Orkin, SH; Hirschhorn, JN. Modifier genes in Mendelian disorders: the example of hemoglobin disorders. Ann N Y Acad Sci., 2010 Dec;1214, 47-56.

[8] Saraf, SL; Molokie, RE; Nouraie, M; Sable, CA; Luchtman-Jones, L; Ensing, GJ, et al. Differences in the clinical and genotypic presentation of sickle cell disease around the world. Paediatr Respir Rev., 2014 Mar;15(1), 4-12. doi: 10.1016/j.prrv.2013.11.003. Epub 2013 Nov 15.

[9] WATSON, J. The significance of the paucity of sickle cells in newborn Negro infants. Am J Med Sci., 1948 Apr; 215(4), 419-23.

[10] Noguchi, CT; Schechter, A. The intracellular polymerization of sickle hemoglobin and its relevance to sickle cell disease, Blood., 1981 Dec; 58(6), 1057-68.

[11] Milton, J; Gordeuk, V; TaylorJ; Gladwin, M; Steinberg, M,Sebastiani, P. Prediction of fetal hemoglobin in sickle cell anemia using an ensemble of genetic risk prediction models. Circ Cardiovasc Genet., 2014, 7, 110-115.

[12] Akinsheye, I; Alsultan, A; Solovieff, N; Ngo, D; Baldwin, CT; Sebastiani, P; et al. Fetal hemoglobin in sickle cell anemia. Blood., 2011 Jul 7, 118(1), 19-27.

[13] Powars, DR; Weiss, JN; Chan, LS; Schroeder, WA. Is there a threshold level of fetal hemoglobin that ameliorates morbidity in sickle cell anemia?. Blood., 1984 Apr;63(4), 921-6.

[14] Sheehan, V; Crosby, J; Sabo, A; Mortier, N; Howrd, T; Muzny, D; et al. Whole exome sequencing identifies Novel genes for Fetal Hemoglobin response to hydroxiuureia in children with Sickle Cell Anemia. PLOS 2014 Oct, vol9 (10): e 110740.

[15] Steinberg, MH; Sebastiani, P; Genetic, modifiers, of, sickle, cell, disease. Am J. Hematol., 2012, 87, 795-803.

[16] Garner, C; Tatu, T; Reittie, JE; Littlewood, T; Darley, J; Cervino, S, et al. Genetic Influences on F cells and other hematologic variables: a twin heritability study. Blood., 2000, 95, 342-346.

[17] Perrine, S; Pace, B; Faller, D. Targeted Fetal Hemoglobin Induction for treatment of Beta Hemoglobinopathies. Hematol Oncol Clin N Am, 2014, 28, 233-248.

[18] Nathan, and, Oski's, Hematology, and, Oncology, of, Infancy, and, Childhood; Eighth, Edition; 2015,; cap, 20; 675-714.

[19] Higgs, DR; Aldridge, BE; Lamb, J; Clegg, JB; Weatherall, DJ; Hayes, RJ, et al. The interaction of alpha-thalassemia and homozygous sickle-cell diseaseN Engl J Med., 1982 Jun 17, 306(24), 1441-6.

[20] Philip, Lanzkowsky. Manual of Pediatric Hematology and Oncology, Fifth Edition , 2011 Chapter 8, 200-246.

[21] Steinberg, MH; Rosenstock, W; Coleman, MB; Adams, JG; Platica, O; Cedeno, M, et al. Effects of thalassemia and microcytosis on the hematologic and vasoocclusive severity of sickle cell anemia. *Blood.*, 1984, 63, 1353–1360.

[22] Kaleyias, J; Mostofi, N; Grant, M; Coleman, C; Luck, L; et al. Severity of obstructive sleep apnea in children with sickle cell disease. *J Pediatr HematolOncol*, 2008, 30, 659-665.

[23] Salles, C; Ramos, RT; Daltro, C; Barral, A; Marinho, JM; Matos, MA. Prevalence of obstructive sleep apnea in children and adolescents with sickle cell anemia. *J Bras Pneumol.*, 2009, 35 (11), 1075-1083.

[24] Lumeng, JC; Chervin, RD. Epidemiology of pediatric obstructive sleep apnea. *Proc Am Thorac Soc.*, 2008, 5(2), 242-252.

[25] Ajulo, SO. The significance of recurrent tonsillitis in sickle cell disease. *Clin Otolaryngol*, 1994, 19, 230-3.

[26] Marcus, CL. Sleep Disordered breathing in children. *Am J Resp Crit Care Med.*, 2001, 164, 16-30.

[27] Quinn, CT; Ahmad, N. Clinical correlates of steady-state oxyhaemoglobin desaturation in children who have sickle cell disease. *Br J Haematol*, 2005, 131, 129-34.

[28] Strauss, T; Sin, S; Marcus, C; Mason, T; McDonough, J; Allen, J; Caboot, J; Bowdre, C; Jawad, A; Smith-Whitley, K; Ohene-Frempong, K; Pack, A; Arens, R. Upper Airway lymphoid tissue size in children with sickle cell disease. 2012. *Chest*, 142 (1), 94-100.

[29] Bandla, H; Splaingard, M. Sleep problems in children with common medical disorders. *Pediatr Clin North Am*, 2004, 51, 201-207.

[30] Valrie, CR; Gil, KM; Redding-Lallinger, R; Daeschner, C. The influence of pain and stress on sleep in children with sickle cell disease. *Children´s health Care*. 2007, 36, 335-353.

[31] Onen, SH; Onen, F; Courpon, P; Dubray, C. How pain and analgesics disturb sleep. *Clin J Pain.*, 2005, 21, 422-431.

[32] Mascarenhas, MI; Loureiro, HC; Ferreira, T; Dias, A. Sleep Pathology characterization in sickle cell disease: a case-control study. *Pediatr Pulmonol.*, 2014 Jul 10. doi: 10.1002/ppul.23074.

[33] Wolf, RB; Kassim, AA; Goodpaster, RL; DeBaun, MR. Nocturnal enuresis in sickle cell disease. *Expert Rev Hematol.*, 2014 Apr, 7(2), 245-54.

[34] Daniels, L; Grant, M; Kothare, S; Dampier, C; Barakat, L. Sleep patterns in Pediatric Sickle cell Disease. *Pediatr Blood Cancer*. 2010, 55, 501-507.

[35] DeBaun, M; Rodeghier, M; CohenR; Kirkham, F; Rosen, C; Roberts, I; et al. Factors predicting future ACS episodes in children with sickle cell anemia. *Am J Hematology*, 2014, vol89, nº11, 212-217.

[36] Rogers, V; Lewin, D; Winnie, G; Geiger-Brown, J. Polysomnographic Characteristics of a referred sample of children with Sickle Cell Disease. *J Clin Sleep Med.*, 20110, vol 6(4), 374-381.

[37] Coelho, A; Dias, A; Morais, A; Nunes, B; Ferreira, E; Picanço, I; et al. Genetic variation in CD36, HBA, NOS3 and VCAM1 is associated with chronic haemolysis level in sickle cell anaemia: a longitudinal study. *Eur J Haematol.*, 2014 Mar, 92(3), 237-43.

[38] Coelho, A; Dias, A; Morais, A; Nunes, B; Faustino, P; Lavinha. Sickle cell disease severity scoring: a yet unsolved problem. *J. Eur J Haematol.*, 2012 Dec, 89(6), 501-2.

[39] Berry, RB; Budhiraja, R; Gottlieb, DJ; Gozal, D; Iber, C; Kapur, VK; et al. Rules for scoring respiratory events in sleep: update of the 2007 AASM Manual for the Scoring of Sleep and Associated Events. Deliberations of the Sleep Apnea Definitions Task Force of the American Academy of Sleep Medicine.

[40] http://www.esst.org/adds/ICSD.pdf, last accessed at March 13, 2015.

[41] Shrivastava, D; Jung, S; Saadat, M; Sirohi, R; Crewson, K. How to interpret the results of a sleep study. *Journal of Community Hospital Internal Medicine Perspectives*, 2014, 4, 24983- http://dx.doi.org/10.3402/jchimp.v4.24983.

In: Sickle Cell Disease
Editor: Marilyn E. Lewis
ISBN: 978-1-63482-828-4

Chapter II

Calcium Handling in Red Blood Cells of Sickle Cell Disease Patients

Anna Bogdanova[1,•]***, Asya Makhro***[1] ***and Lars Kaestner***[2]

[1]Institute of Veterinary Physiology and the Zurich Center for Integrative Human Physiology (ZIHP), University of Zurich, Zurich, Switzerland

[2]Research Center for Molecular Imaging and Screening, Medical School, Institute for Molecular Cell Biology, Saarland University, Homburg/Saar, Germany

Abstract

Precise control over the intracellular free Ca^{2+} level is of key importance for any cell, red blood cells (RBCs) included. Cell fate of erythroid precursor cells, as well as volume, redox state, deformability, aggregability, adherence to the endothelial layer, and membrane stability of circulating RBCs, and as a result RBC longevity, are regulated by Ca^{2+}. Several hereditary forms of hemolytic anemia, including sickle cell disease (SCD), are associated with abnormally high Ca^{2+} uptake, and as a result, Ca^{2+} overload. Multiple organ failure, stroke, and myocardial infarction caused by thrombosis as well as repeated hemolytic and pain

• E-mail: annab@access.uzh.ch.

crises are induced by irreversible polymerization of deoxygenated hemoglobin S in RBCs of these patients. Dehydration of RBCs speed up sickle cell transformation, extensive oxidation and facilitated proteolysis, as well as increased adherence of circulating RBCs to the endothelial layer, substantially contribute to the sickle cell disease manifestation. As all of these processes are driven by the high intraerythrocytic Ca^{2+} levels, inhibition of pathologically high Ca^{2+} uptake would be a powerful therapeutic strategy. Molecular identity of ion channels involved in pathologically high permeability of RBC membranes of patients for Ca^{2+} is a subject of intensive investigation. Among the identified channels are Piezo channels and N-methyl D-aspartate (NMDA) receptors. The contribution of transient voltage receptor channels (TRPCs), voltage-gated calcium channels Cav2.1, and even voltage-dependent anion channels (VDACs) into the Ca^{2+} uptake is currently being debated. This chapter is an overview of the current progress in research in this area followed by an outlook into the potential use of blockers of the cation channels for therapy of SCD patients.

1. Calcium in RBC and Malaria Infection Success

The first reports on reduced susceptibility of RBCs of people with sickle cell traits to malaria date back to the 1950s [3, 23]. Co-localization in the areas with sickle cell trait and malaria prevalence suggest that malaria is a driving force for the preferential evolutionary selection for these otherwise potentially deadly mutations (when reaching homozygosis) in certain areas of the world. Later on, protective features were confirmed for several other hereditary forms of anemia including hemoglobinopathies (α- and β-thalassemia (reviewed in [82]), metabolic disorders (Glucose-6-phosphate dehydrogenase (G6PD) deficiency and pyruvate kinase (PK) deficiency), as well as a number of membrane-related disorders (e.g., Southeast Asian ovalocytosis (band 3 mutation), Duffy antigen variants, glycophorins A and C variant, and complement receptor 1 polymorphism [96, 112]). The advantages provided by these particular polymorphisms, as well as the molecular mechanisms conferring protection against the infection, are not always clear. In order to be protective against malaria one or more of the scenarios should be realized: (i) invasion of the parasite is compromised, (ii) suppression of its growth during the intraerythrocytic stages is achieved, or (iii) phagocytosis/clearance of the infected RBCs is facilitated [164]. A number of glycosylated and sialated integral proteins of the RBC membrane are involved in the interaction with the parasite during the invasion process. Duffi antigen is one of the key players involved in *P. vivax* invasion success whereas glycophorins A and C, and probably band 3 protein, are essential for the successful invasion of *P. falciparum* (reviewed in [36]). Omission of the extracellular Ca^{2+}, or chelation of the intracellular Ca^{2+}, was also shown *ex vivo* to interfere with the RBC invasion of *P. falciparum*, although the exact calcium ions and Ca^{2+}-dependent signalling is unclear [107, 158-160]. Moreover, development of the parasite in RBCs suspended in the Ca^{2+}-free medium is arrested [159].

Phagocytosis of infected RBCs is enhanced in patients with sickle cell trait or β-thalassemia [9], as well as in patients with G6PD deficiency [27]. Moreover, mechanical stability of RBCs with most of the polymorphisms, including sickle cell trait and SCD, may be compromised due to the hemoglobin polymerization triggered by the malaria infection [99, 136]. Furthermore, RBCs resistant to malaria are under conditions of permanent oxidative stress resulting from the hemoglobin variants' instability [56, 117] and abnormally high levels of hyperactivated NADPH oxidases contribute to the oxidative burst in RBCs of SCD patients [61]. Deformability of such RBCs is reduced [12, 117] as the cytoskeleton is disrupted and the cells are dehydrated and oxidized. One more common feature of the majority of gene variances conveying protection to malaria is increased permeability of RBC membranes to Ca^{2+} and/or high intracellular Ca^{2+} levels [19, 25, 53].

Finally, maintenance of the optimal Ca^{2+} levels in the environment and in various compartments of *Plasmodium* has been shown to be pivotal for its survival and growth in the erythrocyte. Interaction between the host's and parasite's Ca^{2+} pools is rather complex (Figure 1).

After the successful invasion, the parasite has to adapt to functioning in the environment with limited free Ca^{2+} availability. Replenishing of the Ca^{2+} endoplasmic reticulum (ER), nuclear and mitochondrial pools requires micromolar levels of Ca^{2+} whereas only 20-30 nM of free Ca2+ ions is available in the cytosol of healthy human RBCs [60]. Increase in the intracellular Ca^{2+} in RBCs to the levels optimal for the *Plasmodium* parasite (40 μM) would result in acute irreversible damage of the host cell. This dilemma is solved as the parasite creates its own microenvironment within the parasitophorous vacuole (Figure 1). It is build of the inside-out oriented RBC plasma membrane with the plasma membrane Ca^{2+} ATPase (PMCA) pumping Ca^{2+} from the RBC cytosol into the vacuole surrounding the parasite [83, 45]. Along with that, Ca^{2+} uptake by the host plasma membrane is increased after the infection [45]. Cytosolic free Ca^{2+} levels at the same time remain largely unchanged [86, 148]. Demand for Ca^{2+} is particularly high at the trophozoit stage of the parasite development [83] when a complex signalling network is established in which mitochondria and ER exchange Ca^{2+} signals in the form of oscillations mediated by the inositol phosphate receptors (IP3R) [59].

Stage-dependent Ca^{2+}-driven signalling pathways are activated and thereby include cGMP-IP3R and cAMP-dependent ones, active in *Plasmodium* controlling its transition from one stage to the other [24, 57]. Blockage of Ca^{2+} oscillations mediating the cross-talk between the plasma membrane, the ER and the mitochondria result in death of the parasite [51]. So far, direct evidence for the existence of this Ca^{2+} signalling network was obtained *ex vivo* in RBCs infected with *Plasmodium* in culture. Recent findings suggest that interference with this Ca^{2+} turnover between the host and *Plasmodium* may indeed be an efficient strategy to achieve resistance to malaria as it was also chosen by natural selection. The association of the polymorphisms in the PMCA4, the dominant isoform of Ca^{2+} pump present in the RBCs, and malaria resistance was reported and confirmed in a large multicenter study [103, 152].

2. Hemoglobinopathies and RBC Membrane Properties

The molecular basis of SCD was identified in 1949 [125]. A point mutation in position 6 of the β globin gene is a cause of polymerization of the deoxygenated hemoglobin S variant [126]. The resulting loss of deformability and rupture of the RBC plasma membrane following the formation of polymerized rod-shaped HbS aggregates was then accepted as a major cause of hemolysis and vaso-occlusive crises [131].

However, most of the time SCD patients are rather asymptomatic. What are the stimuli inducing the sickle cell transformation at the onset of a crisis? The availability of HbS does not change, and the alterations in the oxygenation state of hemoglobin are not always associated with it. In contrast, sickle cell transformation at the onset of a crisis is most likely related to the inflammation or infection followed by an increase in the endothelin-1 (ET-1) and prostaglandin E_2 (PGE_2) levels [65]. Vasoconstriction, occurring upon release of ET-1, invokes an increase in shear stress to which RBCs of patients are exposed [52]. One of the factors crucial for the rapid onset of HbS polymerization is cell volume. Dehydration of RBCs increase the probability for polymerization by 20-40-fold [50]. Dehydration, in turn, is promoted by the up-regulated intracellular free Ca^{2+} levels as it stimulates K^+ loss from the cells via the Gardos channels, and does not occur in a Ca^{2+}-free environment [88].

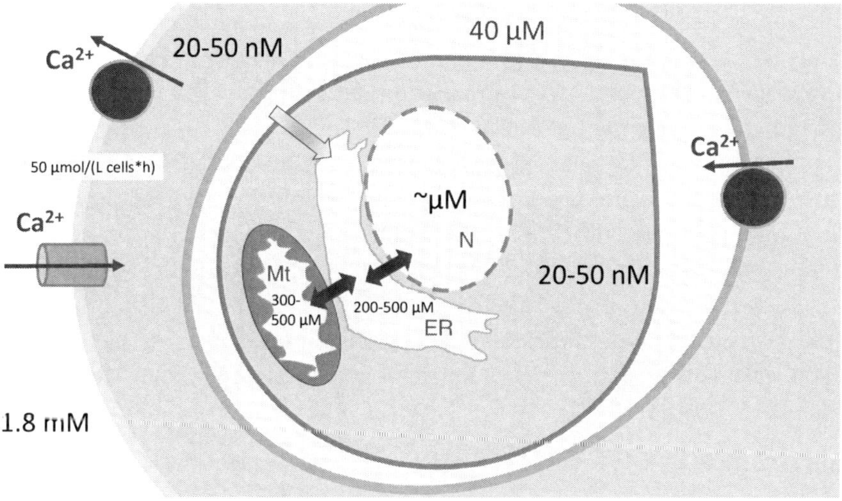

Figure 1. Ca^{2+} in hosting RBC and *Plasmodium* parasite (for comments see the text). N: nucleus, ER: endoplasmic reticulum, Mt: mitochondira. Concentrations given are of free Ca^{2+} ions.

Is there a link between the hemoglobin variant, which is prone to polymerization, its oxygenation, and abnormalities in ion/water balance in RBCs? Oxygen affinity of membrane-bound hemoglobin retained in so-called "pink ghosts" is lower than that of "bulk" cytosolic hemoglobin pool [153]. This hemoglobin functions as an oxygen sensor rather than an oxygen carrier, transferring information to other membrane proteins such as ion transporters. It most likely occurs via the cytoplasmic domain of band 3 protein containing the hemoglobin binding site [156]. Band 3 is one of the most abundant RBC membrane proteins and a key element of the protein complexes participating in docking of the cytoskeletal spectrum network to the membrane (ankyrin and junction complexes [113]). Thus, membrane-bound hemoglobin turns into the active regulator of membrane properties, and *vice versa*, the RBC membrane becomes the regulator of hemoglobin properties, including HbS polymerization.

The following observations suggest that the RBC membrane is a regulator of HbS polymerization, and a bridge between the mutated hemoglobin and the complex abnormalities contributing to the manifestation of SCD. (i) Apart of being capable of binding HbS, band 3 protein is an efficient catalyst for HbS polymerization [137]. (ii) Membrane-bound HbS is making ion transporters sensitive to the changes in its deoxygenation [63]. (iii) Targeted binding of Hb and the products of its degradation to band 3 protein facilitates oxidation and clustering of band 3 protein [94, 161]. (iv) Deoxyhemoglobin competes with glycolytic enzymes for binding to the cytosolic domain of band 3 protein interfering thereby with ATP production [32, 97, 110]. Participation of hemoglobin in control of ion transport in RBCs was directly proven for the K-Cl cotransporter which retained oxygen-sensitivity in "pink ghosts" prepared from SCD-RBCs, retaining membrane-bound hemoglobin fraction, but lost in "white ghosts" deprived of membrane-bound hemoglobin [80]. A number of ion transporters responding to the changes in oxygen availability were shown to interact with band 3-containing protein complexes [14]. Targeted deletion of the key elements of these ankyrin and junction complexes, such as 4.2 protein, result in alteration of a number of ion transporters and dehydration [127].

3. Ca^{2+} in RBCs of SCD Patients

In healthy human RBCs, transmembrane exchange (uptake and extrusion) of Ca^{2+} are balanced at 50 μmol/(Lcells×h) [46, 91]. In RBCs of SCD patients, Ca^{2+} uptake is increased to 300 μmol/(Lcells×h) during the crises associated with sickling [53]. This increase in Ca^{2+} permeability is reversible [90]. Maximal activity of the PMCA in SCD RBCs is lower than that in healthy humans [120]. Because of this shift, in balance between the PMCA and the Ca^{2+} leak components, bulk intracellular calcium content in patients' RBCs increases. Ca^{2+} distribution between the cells in SCD-RBC population and even within single red cells shows marked heterogeneity [49]. During the asymptomatic periods, free Ca^{2+} levels in the cytosol of the SCD-RBCs are maintained low since most of excessive Ca^{2+} is sequestered in the inside-out vesicles within RBCs [89, 132]. This adaptive response reduced K^+ leak through the Gardos channels and interfered with dehydration [122]. Formation of these intracellular Ca^{2+} pools is believed to represent slow stress-driven endocytosis triggered by Ca^{2+} uptake and the following oxidative stress and results in cytoskeletal rearrangements [128, 138, 162, 165]. Despite the fact that ATP depletion induces vesiculation of RBC membrane [155], terminal

ATP deprivation would make Ca^{2+} sequestration in them impossible as the functional Ca^{2+} pump, fueled by the ATP from the cytoplasmic pool, is required to pump Ca^{2+} into the vesicles against the transmembrane Ca^{2+} gradient.

During the crises, Ca^{2+} uptake increases exceeding the intracellular sequestration capacity. Severity of disease manifestation (sickling), is correlated with the Ca^{2+} levels [145] as deoxygenation promotes Ca^{2+} uptake and release of ionized Ca^{2+} from the intracellular proteins (reduction in buffering capacity) [150, 151, 154].

Ex vivo studies revealed that bulk Ca^{2+} levels were the highest in dense populations of SCD cells, decreasing in the medium and light fractions separated on stractan gradient [122]. Recent studies indicated, however, that Ca^{2+} uptake into the SCD-RBCs was dependent on the presence of amino acids (glutamate and glycine) and shear stress while passing through the density gradients as well as on the hemoglobin deoxygenation [67, 154]. These reports question the value of the findings obtained for fully oxygenated cells suspended in amino acids-free buffer. Furthermore, the number of N-methyl D-aspartate (NMDA) receptors, ligand-gated Ca^{2+}-permeable non-selective channels, was shown to be maximal in reticulocytes and young cells, forming the low-density fraction of RBCs of healthy humans [101] and in all RBC fractions of SCD patients [67].

Substantial amounts of young cells and rcticulocytes were dehydrating when passing through the Percoll gradient or cellulose column used to leucodeprive RBCs of SCD patients [67]. Mechanosensitive dehydration could be prevented by pre-treatment with the antagonists of the NMDA receptor memantine or MK-801 [67]. These findings support the earlier observation that reticulocytes and young cells of SCD patients are more susceptible to dehydration and premature clearance than the mature RBCs [18]. Mechanical stress induces cation leakage through the membranes of SCD-RBCs, independent of the oxygenation state of HbS [146], indicating that the existence of both oxygen-dependent and oxygen-independent cation transport pathways are causing cell shrinkage.

Intracellular Ca^{2+} level is not constant, but is dynamically regulated by the alteration in activity of ion channels and the PMCA as well as the buffering capacities of the cytoplasmic proteins. It undergoes permanent fluctuations in each single cell, and the amplitude of these fluctuations is maximal in the vicinity of plasma membrane. Transient bouts of Ca^{2+} uptake cause an increase in free Ca^{2+} levels in the vicinity of the plasma membrane and induces opening of the Ca^{2+} sensitive Gardos channel and anion channels [168–170].

Opening of cation channels occurs in response to the various stimuli including mechanical stimulation, increase in plasma glutamate or pro-inflammatory cytokine levels or deoxygenation. All these factors contributing to the up-regulation of Ca^{2+} levels in RBCs of SCD patients, trigger opening of several cation channels that we term here as P_{sickle}. This term was introduced to describe deoxygenation-induced cation current [90, 100], but this definition might be too narrow taking into account the identity of the contributing ion channels. This transient bout of P_{sickle} activation is followed by deactivation of the channels. Several minutes are then required (at room temperature) for the Ca^{2+} ATPase to restore the Ca^{2+} levels to the "steady state". If stimulation of the channels persists, a new "steady state" is reached. One of the channels involved in these fluctuations is the NMDA receptor mentioned above. This is not the only channel known to contribute to the electrogenic "cation leak" in SCD RBCs known as P_{sickle}. The properties of this transport pathway suggest that it has a compound nature. It is suggested that one component of P_{sickle} triggered by deoxygenation [72, 90] may be represented by Piezo1 [58]. Mutations in this non-selective cation channel are associated with hereditary xerocytosis [167], it is mechano-sensitive [35], and can be inhibited by the tarantula spider toxin GsMTx-4 [10]. The first cell-attached recordings of this channel in RBCs of patients with hereditary xerocytosis are published [7], however comparisons to healthy cells or SCD-RBCs are missing. In a different approach, electrophysiological characterization of the P_{sickle} revealed its sensitivity to GsMTx-4 [100], suggesting that Piezo1 may contribute to P_{sickle}, however, the molecular proof of the involvement of this channel in Ca^{2+} uptake is pending. NMDA receptor is one more candidate to contribute to the P_{sickle} [101]. This receptor is involved in regulation of the intracellular Ca^{2+} in erythroid precursor cells and in the circulating RBCs of healthy subjects and SCD patients [67, 101] Its abundance is abnormally high in all cells of SCD patients, even during asymptomatic periods, increasing further during the hemolytic crises [67]. It is mechano- and oxygen-sensitive in patients' RBCs, and its inhibitor memantine substantially alleviates dehydration and sickling caused by deoxygenation [67]. A putative sensitivity towards GsMTx-4 remains to be tested. Recent findings of Kaestner et al. indicate that apart of TRPC6, an omega-Agatoxin TK-sensitive Ca^{2+}entry associated with the $Ca_V2.1$ [4] may also be involved in the abnormal permeability of SCD-RBCs to Ca^{2+} [77]. This list may be incomplete without Pannexin 1 [95] and a voltage dependent anion channel (VDAC) [21], which under certain conditions can conduct cations and Ca^{2+} in particular [34], may contribute to the cation leakage of RBC membranes of SCD patients. Furthermore, a number of cation channels characterized at the functional level in RBCs, such as the voltage-activated non-selective cation channel [30, 74, 134], a low conductance cation channel [13, 66, 73] or receptor activated channels [48, 76, 116] await molecular identification and clarification of their physiological role in function and fate of the erythroid progenitors and the circulating RBCs. Mature RBCs are not capable of sustaining de novo protein synthesis. Thus, according to current knowledge, the excess of a given ion channel in diseased RBCs is either resulting from its over-expression in erythroid precursor cells or from the disturbed clearance of the channels during the final stages of differentiation and maturation of the circulating cells. Alternatively, post-transcriptional modifications of the channels or the pathological environment (plasma-borne oxidants, cytokines, shear stress due to vasoconstriction, and mechanical damage by the HbS polymers) may result in increased activity whereas the number of channel copies remains unchanged. No differences in expression levels of the subunits of NMDA receptors was found in the *ex vivo* cultures of erythroid precursor cells of SCD patients compared to that in cells of healthy people.

However, the circulating RBCs of the same patients contained 8-10-fold higher numbers of the functional NMDA receptors [67], suggesting that the enrichment occurred at the stage of receptor clearance rather than over-expression.

This is not the only transporter for which the abundance in RBC membranes of patients was shown to exceed that in RBCs of healthy donors. Similar observations were reported for the K-Cl cotransporter [26]. These features, characteristic for immature RBCs in part, reflect the dramatically reduced life span of RBCs in patients with SCD (8-29 days vs. 100-120 days for the cells of healthy donors [108]) and stress erythropoiesis typical for this pathological condition [47]).

The number of copies of NMDA receptors in early erythroid precursors is estimated to be ~300 000 per cells, whereas in young healthy RBCs it drops to ~30 [101]. This number is 10-fold higher in patients in hemolytic crises [67]. One more reason for the incomplete shedding of membrane proteins relates to the abnormally high affinity of HbS to the cytosolic domain of band 3 proteins and deposition of the degraded hemoglobin products at the membrane surface [117, 137]. This mechanical obstacle may impair shedding, making the RBC membrane rigid.

4. Downstream Targets of Intracellular Ca^{2+}

4.1. Metabolism

Fueling the ion pumps is a major source of ATP expenditure in RBCs along with regulatory phosphorylation. Due to the increased "leakiness" of the membranes of SCD-RBCs for cations, ATP hydrolysis by the ion pumps is facilitated in these cells creating conditions of ATP depletion. The resulting AMP accumulation creates the risk of irreversible adenine nucleotide loss via Ca^{2+}-activated AMP to IMP conversion by AMP deaminase. Adenine supplementation helps to prevent ATP depletion [139]. Facilitated Ca^{2+} uptake stimulates the PMCA causing ATP deficiency in SCD-RBCs which is particularly pronounced in the pre-membrane space. ATP in RBCs is highly compartmentalized and the ion pumps are using it from the pre-membrane ATP pools [68]. These "pockets" are formed by ankyrin, spectrin, and the cytosolic domain of band 3 protein, to which the glycolytic proteins (metabolon) are attached [33, 129]. Recruitment of the Ca^{2+}-sensitive protein kinase C alpha (PKCα) to the plasma membrane of SCD-RBCs [54] occurs upon stimulation of Ca^{2+} uptake by deoxygenation and adds to the ATP depletion in the pre-membrane space [5]. ATP deprivation has multiple consequences as dissipation of ion gradients, oxidative stress and cytoskeletal re-arrangements are associated with excessive vesiculation.

4.2. Ion Gradients and Volume

RBCs of patients with SCD are known for their dehydration resulting from massive K^+ loss, which is only partially compensated by the facilitated Na^+ uptake [87]. As mentioned above, patients' cells excessively take up Ca^{2+}, particularly under conditions of mechanical stress, deoxygenation or stimulation with agonist of the NMDA receptors as well as PGE_2 [76, 157]. The source of PGE2 released into the circulation during the crises in SCD patients remains to be identified, and RBCs may take part in it since they were reported to be capable of PGE2 production and release [121]. Increase in free Ca^{2+} level in the cells induced by any of the above-mentioned stimuli above 1 μM triggers opening of the Gardos channel and K+ leak [15]. Oxidative burst triggered by the opening of Ca^{2+}-permeable channels further facilitates leakage of K^+ through the K-Cl cotransporter [1, 67]. Ca^{2+}-driven binding of band 4.2 protein to band 3 [80] down-regulates band 3 transport activity [39], which, however, does not limit K^+ loss after the activation of Gardos channels. Passive Na^+ uptake by the Na/H exchanger is activated by Ca^{2+}-sensitive PKCα-driven phosphorylation [28]. At the same time Na,K-ATPase is inhibited due to the depletion of the pre-membrane ATP pool and phosphorylation catalyzed by PKCα [29]. Deoxygenation results in further suppression of the Na,K-ATPase, which was suggested to be caused by the increase in Mg/ATP ratio [123]. Interestingly, PKCα is also involved in a Ca^{2+}-dependent compensatory activation of the PMCA and suppression of the Gardos channels [54].

Dehydration was chosen as a pharmacological target as a synthetic blocker of Gardos channels Senicapoc (ICA-17043, Icagen) and was used in a clinical trial. The trial was terminated due to the inability of the drug to reduce the occurrence and severity of vaso-occlusive crises and pain syndrome although reduction of hemolysis was observed [8].

4.3. Cytoskeleton Rearrangements and Proteolysis

RBC cytoskeletal stability may be compromised by the Ca^{2+}-calmodulin complex (reviewed in [15]). It down-regulates the adducin capping activity thereby regulating actin filament assembly and, most importantly, reduces affinity of the band 4.1R protein to its interacting partners (band 3, p55, and glycophorin C). This facilitates dissociation of the cytoskeletal spectrin mesh from the membrane and mechanical destabilization of the cell upon shear stress.

High intracellular Ca^{2+} combined with ATP depletion alters tyrosine phosphorylation of RBC membrane proteins [43]. In SCD-RBCs hypophosphorylation of spectrin was observed [44], which is associated with the loss of membrane integrity and the inability to resist mechanical stress [104]. Along with that, PKCα targets including band 4.1R protein, and adducin, were hyperphosphorylated [15, 62].

Ca^{2+} is known to promote band 3 tyrosine phosphorylation [168] at Tyr 9 and 21. This regulatory phosphorylation causes displacement of the glycolytic enzymes from the cytosolic domain of band 3, which also occurs upon binding of deoxygenated hemoglobin to it [31, 32].

Hyperphosphorylation of band 3 at tyrosine residues was reported in cells of SCD patients [149]. *In vitro* tyrosine phosphorylation was shown to decrease its affinity to ankyrin, causing band 3 diffusion and clustering [55]. Hyperphosphorylation of band 3 produces abnormal membrane topology resembling that of echinocytes [55]. The molecular mechanism behind Ca^{2+}-driven tyrosine phosphorylation is unknown, but may be related to the oxidative burst that down-regulates the function of SHP-1 tyrosine phosphatase [22]. Interestingly, abnormally high levels of band 3 phosphorylation could not be correlated to the age of SCD-RBCs [70].

One of the most prominent effects of intracellular Ca^{2+} overload in RBCs is μ-calpain activation followed by proteolysis of various proteins including cytoskeletal elements, band 3 protein, PMCA and hemoglobin [109]. By cleaving hemoglobin, μ-calpain contributes to the oxidative damage and formation of Heinz bodies [114]. Calpain inhibitors were suggested as a drug for SCD treatment, since a marked improvement in RBC morphology was observed in the animal model of SCD [41].

4.4. Redox State

Oxidation is a hallmark of early RBC senescence [6]. Hemoglobin auto-oxidation and accumulation of degraded hemoglobin aggregates (Heinz bodies) at the membrane surface facilitates condition of permanent oxidative stress, which is obviously Ca^{2+}-independent ([133] for review). However, increase in the intracellular Ca^{2+} in SCD-RBCs upon stimulation of the NMDA receptors was shown to induce oxidative stress, which could be abolished by the receptor antagonist [67]. Recently a new Ca^{2+}-sensitive source of superoxide anion production was discovered, which appeared to be over-represented in membranes of SCD-RBCs, namely NADPH oxidases (NOXes) [61]. Several isoforms of this protein family were reported to be present in RBCs, of which NOX5 is directly stimulated by Ca^{2+} whereas the other one, NOX1, is regulated by Ca^{2+}-dependent conventional PKC isoforms and Rac kinase [61]. In addition to NOXes activity, intracellular Ca^{2+} controls NO production by the endothelial NO synthase (eNOS) present in RBC membranes of rodents and humans [81, 102]. Chronic hyperactivation of eNOS results in arginine deprivation and a switch from NO to $O_2^{\bullet-}$ generation [111]. Plasma arginine levels were reported to be low in children with SCD during the vaso-occlusive crises indicating up-regulation of its utilization by NOS [115]. Arginine therapy used in the animal model of SCD successfully reduced oxidative stress and hemolysis [79]. Being a poor oxidant, superoxide anion produced by NOXes joins Haver-Weiss reactions and is transformed into H_2O_2 by superoxide dismutase. The resulting oxidants are produced at the membrane surface and oxidize membrane proteins (including band 3 [106], [6, 98]) and lipids [130], [69], [130] [166] and triggers rapid clearance of the SCD-RBCs from the circulation. Both *in vitro* studies and clinical trials showed that antioxidant supplementation reduced formation of sickle cells [64] and lowered frequency of vaso-occlusive crises [124].

4.5. RBC Aggregation, Thrombosis and Clearance

Several factors contribute to the repeated vaso-occlusive crises characteristic for SCD. Some of these factors are directly related to the RBC abnormalities, some are associated with other cell types such as platelets, monocytes, and vascular endothelium.

Increased aggregability of RBCs to each other and to the endothelium is associated with phosphatidylserine (PS) exposure to the outer leaflet of the RBC membrane. When exposed, PS interacts with thrombospondin receptors at the endothelial cells increasing RBC adhesion to the endothelium [105]. Furthermore, PS exposure during the deoxygenation triggers erythrocyte's recognition by peripheral blood monocytes [140] and facilitates their removal from the circulation. PS exposure is facilitated by ATP depletion [139, 143], and may be caused by Ca^{2+} overload [16, 42], although some reports are stating that it is not always the case [118]. There are four potent mechanisms regulated by Ca^{2+} involved in Ca^{2+}-induced PS exposure: (i) the competition for ATP fuel between ion pumps and PS flippase in premembrane space, (ii) direct inhibition of PS flippase by Ca^{2+} ions [142, 163], (iii) activation of the scramblase and (iv) Secondary PKCα-mediated pathway [42].

Apart from increased adherence to the endothelial cells, inter-cellular interaction between the RBCs is promoted by stimulating induced Ca^{2+} uptake such as lysophosphatidic acid (LPA) or PGE_2 [75, 76, 144]. Increase in PGE_2 in plasma of patients with SCD during vaso-occlusive crises [65] is therefore promoting RBC aggregation.

Vaso-occlusive crises in SCD patients have a very complex pathology involving several types of cells, with endothelial cells and platelets showing the most prominent abnormalities (for review see [40]). Cross-talk mechanisms between the RBCs containing the mutated beta globin chain and the other cells remain largely unknown. Overview of the processes involved in vaso-occlusive activity is out of the scope of this chapter apart from the Ca^{2+}-dependent events. Mechanical rigidity of dehydrated and, particularly, "sickled" RBCs, hemolytic activity and release of free hemoglobin and other cytosolic components as well as release of vesicles or microparticles are the possible "messengers" contributing to the platelet activation. Up-regulation of the intracellular Ca^{2+} levels trigger extensive formation of endo- and exo-vesicles, and is likely to promote thereby inflammatory and pro-thrombotic activity. Whether these microparticles actively participate in platelet activation and inflammatory response remains to be established.

4.6. Similarities between SCD, Thalassemia and G6PD Deficiency

Ca^{2+} overload leaves typical fingerprints shared by all RBC pathologies including thalassemia, favism (G6PD deficiency), familiar PFK deficiency and several other forms of rare anemia [135]. Characteristic calpain-induced protein cleavage was reported in the RBCs of patients with G6PD-deficiency [37, 114] and β-thalassemia [147]. Oxidative stress and oxidative damage are known to contribute to the premature clearance of RBCs in patients with favism [39] [71] and thalassemia [2]. Membrane instability arises from oxidation and cleavage of the cytoskeletal components such as spectrin, ankyrin, protein 4.1 and band 3 [2, 37, 141]. High levels of band 3 tyrosine phosphorylation were observed in patients with hemoglobinopathies (HbS, HbC and β-thalassemia) [149]. Potassium loss from the cells secondary to Ca^{2+} accumulation and oxidation is a cause of RBC dehydration [38, 119]. Facilitated PS exposure is another feature characteristic for the congenital RBC disorders associated with high intracellular Ca^{2+}, such as thalassemia [84] [20].

5. Ca^{2+} Influx Pathways As Targets for Therapy

It appears that Ca^{2+} is indeed a puppeteer, setting in motion multiple processes forming the complex etiology of SCD. Increase in Ca^{2+} levels is mediated by the activation of multiple ion channels permeable for Ca^{2+} in response to inflammation (PGE_2), shear stress, and deoxygenation. Transient increase in free Ca^{2+} levels in the pre-membrane space results in RBC shrinkage, activation of caspases, oxidative burst, re-programming of the glycolytic enzymes and re-profiling of phosphorylation state of multiple proteins. Gaining control of Ca^{2+} uptake will enable it to take over the fate of RBCs, increasing their stability and reducing their adherence to the endothelium [75, 144]. Out of the Ca^{2+} uptake pathways listed above, Piezo1 and the NMDA-receptor are the most promising candidates for pharmacological intervention. Unfortunately, for Piezo1 no selective non-toxic inhibitors are currently available. The blockers used *in vitro* (e.g., ruthenium red or Gd^{3+}) are not entirely specific and inhibit a number of other vital essentials [35]. Fairly specific blockers like GsMTx-4 [10] are expected to have severe side effects due to the systemic importance of Piezo1 [11, 92]. In contrast to that, pharmacological advances in the field of the NMDA receptors' antagonists design are impressive. Several generations of several classes of drugs have been produced and tested in clinical trials. Memantine is the compound that is proven to have the best benefits-to-risks ratio [93]. Memantine was proven to effectively block deoxygenation-induced Ca^{2+} uptake into the RBCs of SCD patients *in vitro*. Rehydration and decrease in oxidation were observed in response to memantine application [67]. Further benefits of using such a therapeutic strategy rise from the action of the NMDA receptor antagonist on the receptors expressed in the circulating platelets [78], immune competent cells [17], and macrophages [85]. Thus, promotion of survival of RBCs and improvement of rheological properties of RBCs of SCD patients are expected to occur along with reduction in platelet activity and suppression of inflammation. The outcome of the clinical trial, in which memantine will be used for treatment of a small cohort of SCD patients at the University Hospital of Zurich, will reveal if the strategy proven beneficial *ex vivo* will be effective *in vivo*.

References

[1] Adragna, N. C. and Lauf, P. K. (1997) Oxidative activation of K-Cl cotransport by diamide in erythrocytes from humans with red cell disorders, and from several other mammalian species. *The Journal of membrane biology,* 155, 207-217.

[2] Advani, R., Sorenson, S., Shinar, E., Lande, W., Rachmilewitz, E. and Schrier, S.L. (1992) Characterization and comparison of the red blood cell membrane damage in severe human alpha- and beta-thalassemia. *Blood,* 79, 1058-1063.

[3] Allison, A. C. (1954) Protection afforded by sickle-cell trait against subtertian malareal infection. *British medical journal,* 1, 290-294.

[4] Andrews, D. A., Yang, L. and Low, P. S. (2002) Phorbol ester stimulates a protein kinase C-mediated agatoxin-TK-sensitive calcium permeability pathway in human red blood cells. *Blood,* 100, 3392-3399.

[5] Apovo, M., Gascard, P., Rhoda, M. D., Beuzard, Y. and Giraud, F. (1989) Alteration in protein kinase C activity and subcellular distribution in sickle erythrocytes. *Biochimica et biophysica acta,* 984, 26-32.

[6] Arashiki, N., Kimata, N., Manno, S., Mohandas, N. and Takakuwa, Y. (2013) Membrane peroxidation and methemoglobin formation are both necessary for band 3 clustering: mechanistic insights into human erythrocyte senescence. *Biochemistry,* 52, 5760-5769.

[7] Archer, N. M., Shmukler, B. E., Andolfo, I., Vandorpe, D. H., Gnanasambandam, R., Higgins, J. M., Rivera, A., Fleming, M. D., Sachs, F., Gottlieb, P. A., Iolascon, A., Brugnara, C., Alper, S. L. and Nathan, D. G. (2014) Hereditary xerocytosis revisited. *American journal of hematology,* 89, 1142-1146.

[8] Ataga, K. I., Reid, M., Ballas, S. K., Yasin, Z., Bigelow, C., James, L. S., Smith, W. R., Galacteros, F., Kutlar, A., Hull, J. H., Stocker, J. W. and Investigators, I.C.A.S. (2011) Improvements in haemolysis and indicators of erythrocyte survival do not correlate with acute vaso-occlusive crises in patients with sickle cell disease: a phase III randomized, placebo-controlled, double-blind study of the Gardos channel blocker senicapoc (ICA-17043). *British journal of haematology,* 153, 92-104.

[9] Ayi, K., Turrini, F., Piga, A. and Arese, P. (2004) Enhanced phagocytosis of ring-parasitized mutant erythrocytes: a common mechanism that may explain protection against falciparum malaria in sickle trait and beta-thalassemia trait. *Blood,* 104, 3364-3371.

[10] Bae, C., Sachs, F. and Gottlieb, P. A. (2011) The mechanosensitive ion channel Piezo1 is inhibited by the peptide GsMTx4. *Biochemistry,* 50, 6295-6300.

[11] Bagriantsev, S. N., Gracheva, E. O. and Gallagher, P. G. (2014) Piezo proteins: regulators of mechanosensation and other cellular processes. *The Journal of biological chemistry,* 289, 31673-31681.

[12] Barodka, V. M., Nagababu, E., Mohanty, J. G., Nyhan, D., Berkowitz, D. E., Rifkind, J. M. and Strouse, J. J. (2014) New insights provided by a comparison of impaired deformability with erythrocyte oxidative stress for sickle cell disease. *Blood cells, molecules and diseases,* 52, 230-235.

[13] Bennekou, P. and Christophersen, P. (1988) The occurance of a low conductance channel in the human red cell. *Acta Physiol. Scand.,* 13, S73.

[14] Bogdanova, A., Berenbrink, M. and Nikinmaa, M. (2009) Oxygen-dependent ion transport in erythrocytes. *Acta physiologica,* 195, 305-319.

[15] Bogdanova, A., Makhro, A., Wang, J., Lipp, P. and Kaestner, L. (2013) Calcium in red blood cells-a perilous balance. *International journal of molecular sciences,* 14, 9848-9872.

[16] Bogitsh, B. J. and Carter, O. S. (1977) Developmental studies on the digestive tract of schistosomules (Schistosoma mansoni) grown in vitro. I. Ultrastructure. *Transactions of the American Microscopical Society,* 96, 219-227.

[17] Boldyrev, A. A., Bryushkova, E. A. and Vladychenskaya, E. A. (2012) NMDA receptors in immune competent cells. *Biochemistry. Biokhimiia,* 77, 128-134.

[18] Bookchin, R. M., Ortiz, O. E. and Lew, V. L. (1991) Evidence for a direct reticulocyte origin of dense red cells in sickle cell anemia. *The Journal of clinical investigation,* 87, 113-124.

[19] Bookchin, R. M., Ortiz, O. E., Shalev, O., Tsurel, S., Rachmilewitz, E. A., Hockaday, A. and Lew, V. L. (1988) Calcium transport and ultrastructure of red cells in beta-thalassemia intermedia. *Blood,* 72, 1602-1607.

[20] Borenstain-Ben Yashar, V., Barenholz, Y., Hy-Am, E., Rachmilewitz, E. A. and Eldor, A. (1993) Phosphatidylserine in the outer leaflet of red blood cells from beta-thalassemia patients may explain the chronic hypercoagulable state and thrombotic episodes. *American journal of hematology,* 44, 63-65.

[21] Bouyer, G., Cueff, A., Egee, S., Kmiecik, J., Maksimova, Y., Glogowska, E., Gallagher, P. G. and Thomas, S. L. (2011) Erythrocyte peripheral type benzodiazepine receptor/voltage-dependent anion channels are upregulated by Plasmodium falciparum. *Blood,* 118, 2305-2312.

[22] Bragadin, M., Ion-Popa, F., Clari, G. and Bordin, L. (2007) SHP-1 tyrosine phosphatase in human erythrocytes. *Annals of the New York Academy of Sciences,* 1095, 193-203.

[23] Brain, P. (1952) The sickle cell trait; its clinical significance. *South African medical journal = Suid-Afrikaanse tydskrif vir geneeskunde,* 26, 925-928.

[24] Brochet, M., Collins, M. O., Smith, T. K., Thompson, E., Sebastian, S., Volkmann, K., Schwach, F., Chappell, L., Gomes, A. R., Berriman, M., Rayner, J. C., Baker, D. A., Choudhary, J. and Billker, O. (2014) Phosphoinositide metabolism links cGMP-dependent protein kinase G to essential Ca(2)(+) signals at key decision points in the life cycle of malaria parasites. *PLoS biology,* 12, e1001806.

[25] Bruce, L. J., Ring, S. M., Ridgwell, K., Reardon, D. M., Seymour, C. A., Van Dort, H. M., Low, P. S. and Tanner, M. J. (1999) South-east asian ovalocytic (SAO) erythrocytes have a cold sensitive cation leak: implications for in vitro studies on stored SAO red cells. *Biochimica et biophysica acta,* 1416, 258-270.

[26] Brugnara, C., Bunn, H. F. and Tosteson, D. C. (1986) Regulation of erythrocyte cation and water content in sickle cell anemia. *Science,* 232, 388-390.

[27] Cappadoro, M., Giribaldi, G., O'Brien, E., Turrini, F., Mannu, F., Ulliers, D., Simula, G., Luzzatto, L. and Arese, P. (1998) Early phagocytosis of glucose-6-phosphate dehydrogenase (G6PD)-deficient erythrocytes parasitized by Plasmodium falciparum may explain malaria protection in G6PD deficiency. *Blood,* 92, 2527-2534.

[28] Ceolotto, G., Sartori, M., Felice, M., Clari, G., Bordin, L. and Semplicini, A. (1999) Effect of protein kinase C and insulin on Na+/H+ exchange in red blood cells of essential hypertensives. *Journal of human hypertension,* 13, 321-327.

[29] Cheng, X. J., Hoog, J. O., Nairn, A. C., Greengard, P. and Aperia, A. (1997) Regulation of rat Na(+)-K(+)-ATPase activity by PKC is modulated by state of phosphorylation of Ser-943 by PKA. *The American journal of physiology,* 273, C1981-1986.

[30] Christophersen, P. and Bennekou, P. (1991) Evidence for a voltage-gated, non-selective cation channel in the human red cell membrane. *Biochimica et biophysica acta,* 1065, 103-106.

[31] Chu, H., Breite, A., Ciraolo, P., Franco, R. S. and Low, P. S. (2008) Characterization of the deoxyhemoglobin binding site on human erythrocyte band 3: implications for O2 regulation of erythrocyte properties. *Blood,* 111, 932-938.

[32] Chu, H. and Low, P. S. (2006) Mapping of glycolytic enzyme-binding sites on human erythrocyte band 3. *The Biochemical journal,* 400, 143-151.

[33] Chu, H., Puchulu-Campanella, E., Galan, J. A., Tao, W. A., Low, P. S. and Hoffman, J. F. (2012) Identification of cytoskeletal elements

enclosing the ATP pools that fuel human red blood cell membrane cation pumps. *Proceedings of the National Academy of Sciences of the United States of America,* 109, 12794-12799.

[34] Colombini, M. (2012) VDAC structure, selectivity, and dynamics. *Biochimica et biophysica acta,* 1818, 1457-1465.

[35] Coste, B., Mathur, J., Schmidt, M., Earley, T. J., Ranade, S., Petrus, M. J., Dubin, A. E. and Patapoutian, A. (2010) Piezo1 and Piezo2 are essential components of distinct mechanically activated cation channels. *Science,* 330, 55-60.

[36] Cowman, A. F. and Crabb, B. S. (2006) Invasion of red blood cells by malaria parasites. *Cell,* 124, 755-766.

[37] Damonte, G., Guida, L., Sdraffa, A., Benatti, U., Melloni, E., Forteleoni, G., Meloni, T., Carafoli, E. and De Flora, A. (1992) Mechanisms of perturbation of erythrocyte calcium homeostasis in favism. *Cell calcium,* 13, 649-658.

[38] De Flora, A., Benatti, U., Guida, L., Forteleoni, G. and Meloni, T. (1985) Favism: disordered erythrocyte calcium homeostasis. *Blood,* 66, 294-297.

[39] De Flora, A., Morelli, A., Grasso, M., Forteleoni, G. and Meloni, T. (1987) Alterations of red blood cell proteolysis in favism. *Biomedica biochimica acta,* 46, S184-189.

[40] De Franceschi, L., Cappellini, M. D. and Olivieri, O. (2011) Thrombosis and sickle cell disease. *Seminars in thrombosis and hemostasis,* 37, 226-236.

[41] De Franceschi, L., Franco, R. S., Bertoldi, M., Brugnara, C., Matte, A., Siciliano, A., Wieschhaus, A. J., Chishti, A. H. and Joiner, C. H. (2013) Pharmacological inhibition of calpain-1 prevents red cell dehydration and reduces Gardos channel activity in a mouse model of sickle cell disease. *FASEB journal: official publication of the Federation of American Societies for Experimental Biology,* 27, 750-759.

[42] de Jong, K., Rettig, M. P., Low, P. S. and Kuypers, F. A. (2002) Protein kinase C activation induces phosphatidylserine exposure on red blood cells. *Biochemistry,* 41, 12562-12567.

[43] Dekkers, D. W., Comfurius, P., Vuist, W. M., Billheimer, J. T., Dicker, I., Weiss, H. J., Zwaal, R. F. and Bevers, E. M. (1998) Impaired Ca2+-induced tyrosine phosphorylation and defective lipid scrambling in erythrocytes from a patient with Scott syndrome: a study using an inhibitor for scramblase that mimics the defect in Scott syndrome. *Blood,* 91, 2133-2138.

[44] Delaunay, J., Galand, C. and Boivin, P. (1982) Erythrocyte membrane phosphorylation in sickle cell disease. *Nouvelle revue francaise d'hematologie,* 24, 227-230.

[45] Desai, S. A., McCleskey, E. W., Schlesinger, P. H. and Krogstad, D. J. (1996) A novel pathway for Ca++ entry into Plasmodium falciparum-infected blood cells. *The American journal of tropical medicine and hygiene,* 54, 464-470.

[46] Desai, S. A., Schlesinger, P. H. and Krogstad, D. J. (1991) Physiologic rate of carrier-mediated Ca2+ entry matches active extrusion in human erythrocytes. *The Journal of general physiology,* 98, 349-364.

[47] Duits, A. J., Rojer, R. A., van Endt, T., MacGillavry, M. R., ten Cate, H., Brandjes, D. P. and Schnog, J. B. (2003) Erythropoiesis and serum sVCAM-1 levels in adults with sickle cell disease. *Annals of hematology,* 82, 171-174.

[48] Duranton, C., Huber, S. M. and Lang, F. (2002) Oxidation induces a Cl(-)-dependent cation conductance in human red blood cells. *The Journal of physiology,* 539, 847-855.

[49] Eaton, J. W., Skelton, T. D., Swofford, H. S., Kolpin, C. E. and Jacob, H. S. (1973) Elevated erythrocyte calcium in sickle cell disease. *Nature,* 246, 105-106.

[50] Eaton, W. A. and Hofrichter, J. (1990) Sickle cell hemoglobin polymerization. *Advances in protein chemistry,* 40, 63-279.

[51] Enomoto, M., Kawazu, S., Kawai, S., Furuyama, W., Ikegami, T., Watanabe, J. and Mikoshiba, K. (2012) Blockage of spontaneous Ca2+ oscillation causes cell death in intraerythrocitic Plasmodium falciparum. *PloS one,* 7, e39499.

[52] Ergul, S., Brunson, C. Y., Hutchinson, J., Tawfik, A., Kutlar, A., Webb, R. C. and Ergul, A. (2004) Vasoactive factors in sickle cell disease: in vitro evidence for endothelin-1-mediated vasoconstriction. *American journal of hematology,* 76, 245-251.

[53] Etzion, Z., Tiffert, T., Bookchin, R. M. and Lew, V. L. (1993) Effects of deoxygenation on active and passive Ca2+ transport and on the cytoplasmic Ca2+ levels of sickle cell anemia red cells. *The Journal of clinical investigation,* 92, 2489-2498.

[54] Fathallah, H., Sauvage, M., Romero, J. R., Canessa, M. and Giraud, F. (1997) Effects of PKC alpha activation on Ca2+ pump and K(Ca) channel in deoxygenated sickle cells. *The American journal of physiology,* 273, C1206-1214.

[55] Ferru, E., Giger, K., Pantaleo, A., Campanella, E., Grey, J., Ritchie, K., Vono, R., Turrini, F. and Low, P. S. (2011) Regulation of membrane-cytoskeletal interactions by tyrosine phosphorylation of erythrocyte band 3. *Blood,* 117, 5998-6006.

[56] Friedman, M. J. (1979) Oxidant damage mediates variant red cell resistance to malaria. *Nature,* 280, 245-247.

[57] Furuyama, W., Enomoto, M., Mossaad, E., Kawai, S., Mikoshiba, K. and Kawazu, S. (2014) An interplay between 2 signaling pathways: melatonin-cAMP and IP3-Ca2+ signaling pathways control intraerythrocytic development of the malaria parasite Plasmodium falciparum. *Biochemical and biophysical research communications,* 446, 125-131.

[58] Gallagher, P. G. (2013) Disorders of red cell volume regulation. *Current opinion in hematology,* 20, 201-207.

[59] Gazarini, M. L. and Garcia, C. R. (2004) The malaria parasite mitochondrion senses cytosolic Ca2+ fluctuations. *Biochemical and biophysical research communications,* 321, 138-144.

[60] Gazarini, M. L., Thomas, A. P., Pozzan, T. and Garcia, C. R. (2003) Calcium signaling in a low calcium environment: how the intracellular malaria parasite solves the problem. *The Journal of cell biology,* 161, 103-110.

[61] George, A., Pushkaran, S., Konstantinidis, D. G., Koochaki, S., Malik, P., Mohandas, N., Zheng, Y., Joiner, C. H. and Kalfa, T. A. (2013) Erythrocyte NADPH oxidase activity modulated by Rac GTPases, PKC, and plasma cytokines contributes to oxidative stress in sickle cell disease. *Blood,* 121, 2099-2107.

[62] George, A., Pushkaran, S., Li, L., An, X., Zheng, Y., Mohandas, N., Joiner, C. H. and Kalfa, T. A. (2010) Altered phosphorylation of cytoskeleton proteins in sickle red blood cells: the role of protein kinase C, Rac GTPases, and reactive oxygen species. *Blood cells, molecules and diseases,* 45, 41-45.

[63] Gibson, J. S. and Ellory, J. C. (2002) Membrane transport in sickle cell disease. *Blood cells, molecules and diseases,* 28, 303-314.

[64] Gibson, X. A., Shartava, A., McIntyre, J., Monteiro, C. A., Zhang, Y., Shah, A., Campbell, N. F. and Goodman, S. R. (1998) The efficacy of reducing agents or antioxidants in blocking the formation of dense cells and irreversibly sickled cells in vitro. *Blood,* 91, 4373-4378.

[65] Graido-Gonzalez, E., Doherty, J. C., Bergreen, E. W., Organ, G., Telfer, M. and McMillen, M. A. (1998) Plasma endothelin-1, cytokine, and

prostaglandin E2 levels in sickle cell disease and acute vaso-occlusive sickle crisis. *Blood,* 92, 2551-2555.

[66] Grygorczyk, R. and Schwarz, W. (1983) Properties of the CA2+-activated K+ conductance of human red cells as revealed by the patch-clamp technique. *Cell calcium,* 4, 499-510.

[67] Hanggi, P., Makhro, A., Gassmann, M., Schmugge, M., Goede, J. S., Speer, O. and Bogdanova, A. (2014) Red blood cells of sickle cell disease patients exhibit abnormally high abundance of N-methyl D-aspartate receptors mediating excessive calcium uptake. *British journal of haematology,* 167, 252-264.

[68] Hoffman, J. F., Dodson, A. and Proverbio, F. (2009) On the functional use of the membrane compartmentalized pool of ATP by the Na+ and Ca++ pumps in human red blood cell ghosts. *The Journal of general physiology,* 134, 351-361.

[69] Jain, S. K. and Shohet, S. B. (1984) A novel phospholipid in irreversibly sickled cells: evidence for in vivo peroxidative membrane damage in sickle cell disease. *Blood,* 63, 362-367.

[70] Johnson, R. M., Dzandu, J. K. and Warth, J. A. (1986) The phosphoproteins of the sickle erythrocyte membrane. *Archives of biochemistry and biophysics,* 244, 202-210.

[71] Johnson, R. M., Ravindranath, Y., ElAlfy, M. S. and Goyette, G., Jr. (1994) Oxidant damage to erythrocyte membrane in glucose-6-phosphate dehydrogenase deficiency: correlation with in vivo reduced glutathione concentration and membrane protein oxidation. *Blood,* 83, 1117-1123.

[72] Joiner, C. H. (1993) Cation transport and volume regulation in sickle red blood cells. *The American journal of physiology,* 264, C251-270.

[73] Kaestner, L. and Bernhardt, I. (2002) Ion channels in the human red blood cell membrane: their further investigation and physiological relevance. *Bioelectrochemistry,* 55, 71-74.

[74] Kaestner, L., Christophersen, P., Bernhardt, I. and Bennekou, P. (2000) The non-selective voltage-activated cation channel in the human red blood cell membrane: reconciliation between two conflicting reports and further characterisation. *Bioelectrochemistry,* 52, 117-125.

[75] Kaestner, L., Steffen, P., Nguyen, D. B., Wang, J., Wagner-Britz, L., Jung, A., Wagner, C. and Bernhardt, I. (2012) Lysophosphatidic acid induced red blood cell aggregation in vitro. *Bioelectrochemistry,* 87, 89-95.

[76] Kaestner, L., Tabellion, W., Lipp, P. and Bernhardt, I. (2004) Prostaglandin E2 activates channel-mediated calcium entry in human erythrocytes: an indication for a blood clot formation supporting process. *Thrombosis and haemostasis,* 92, 1269-1272.

[77] Kaestner, L., Wang, J., Wagner-Britz, L., Bogdanova, A., Wiesen K. and Tian, Q. (2013) Lysophosphatidic acid signalling in red cells. *Biophys. J.,* 104, 610a-611a.

[78] Kalev-Zylinska, M. L., Green, T. N., Morel-Kopp, M. C., Sun, P. P., Park, Y. E., Lasham, A., During, M. J. and Ward, C. M. (2014) N-methyl-D-aspartate receptors amplify activation and aggregation of human platelets. *Thrombosis research,* 133, 837-847.

[79] Kaul, D. K., Zhang, X., Dasgupta, T. and Fabry, M. E. (2008) Arginine therapy of transgenic-knockout sickle mice improves microvascular function by reducing non-nitric oxide vasodilators, hemolysis, and oxidative stress. *American journal of physiology. Heart and circulatory physiology,* 295, H39-47.

[80] Khan, A. I., Drew, C., Ball, S. E., Ball, V., Ellory, J. C. and Gibson, J. S. (2004) Oxygen dependence of K(+)-Cl- cotransport in human red cell ghosts and sickle cells. *Bioelectrochemistry,* 62, 141-146.

[81] Kleinbongard, P., Schulz, R., Rassaf, T., Lauer, T., Dejam, A., Jax, T., Kumara, I., Gharini, P., Kabanova, S., Ozuyaman, B., Schnurch, H. G., Godecke, A., Weber, A. A., Robenek, M., Robenek, H., Bloch, W., Rosen, P. and Kelm, M. (2006) Red blood cells express a functional endothelial nitric oxide synthase. *Blood,* 107, 2943-2951.

[82] Kotila, T. R. (2012) Thalassaemia is a tropical disease. *Annals of Ibadan postgraduate medicine,* 10, 11-15.

[83] Kramer, R. and Ginsburg, H. (1991) Calcium transport and compartment analysis of free and exchangeable calcium in Plasmodium falciparum-infected red blood cells. *The Journal of protozoology,* 38, 594-601.

[84] Kuypers, F. A., Yuan, J., Lewis, R. A., Snyder, L. M., Kiefer, C. R., Bunyaratvej, A., Fucharoen, S., Ma, L., Styles, L., de Jong, K. and Schrier, S. L. (1998) Membrane phospholipid asymmetry in human thalassemia. *Blood,* 91, 3044-3051.

[85] Lee, Y. S., Lee, S. J., Seo, K. W., Bae, J. U., Park, S. Y. and Kim, C. D. (2013) Homocysteine induces COX-2 expression in macrophages through ROS generated by NMDA receptor-calcium signaling pathways. *Free radical research,* 47, 422-431.

[86] Leida, M. N., Mahoney, J. R. and Eaton, J. W. (1981) Intraerythrocytic plasmodial calcium metabolism. *Biochemical and biophysical research communications,* 103, 402-406.

[87] Lew, V. L. and Bookchin, R. M. (2005) Ion transport pathology in the mechanism of sickle cell dehydration. *Physiological reviews,* 85, 179-200.

[88] Lew, V. L., Etzion, Z. and Bookchin, R. M. (2002) Dehydration response of sickle cells to sickling-induced Ca(++) permeabilization. *Blood,* 99, 2578-2585.

[89] Lew, V. L., Hockaday, A., Sepulveda, M. I., Somlyo, A. P., Somlyo, A. V., Ortiz, O. E. and Bookchin, R. M. (1985) Compartmentalization of sickle-cell calcium in endocytic inside-out vesicles. *Nature,* 315, 586-589.

[90] Lew, V. L., Ortiz, O. E. and Bookchin, R. M. (1997) Stochastic nature and red cell population distribution of the sickling-induced Ca2+ permeability. *The Journal of clinical investigation,* 99, 2727-2735.

[91] Lew, V. L., Tsien, R. Y., Miner, C. and Bookchin, R. M. (1982) Physiological [Ca2+]i level and pump-leak turnover in intact red cells measured using an incorporated Ca chelator. *Nature,* 298, 478-481.

[92] Li, J., Hou, B., Tumova, S., Muraki, K., Bruns, A., Ludlow, M. J., Sedo, A., Hyman, A. J., McKeown, L., Young, R. S., Yuldasheva, N. Y., Majeed, Y., Wilson, L. A., Rode, B., Bailey, M. A., Kim, H. R., Fu, Z., Carter, D. A., Bilton, J., Imrie, H., Ajuh, P., Dear, T. N., Cubbon, R. M., Kearney, M. T., Prasad, K. R., Evans, P. C., Ainscough, J. F. and Beech, D. J. (2014) Piezo1 integration of vascular architecture with physiological force. *Nature,* 515, 279-282.

[93] Lipton, S. A. (2005) The molecular basis of memantine action in Alzheimer's disease and other neurologic disorders: low-affinity, uncompetitive antagonism. *Current Alzheimer research,* 2, 155-165.

[94] Liu, S. C., Yi, S. J., Mehta, J. R., Nichols, P. E., Ballas, S. K., Yacono, P. W., Golan, D. E. and Palek, J. (1996) Red cell membrane remodeling in sickle cell anemia. Sequestration of membrane lipids and proteins in Heinz bodies. *The Journal of clinical investigation,* 97, 29-36.

[95] Locovei, S., Bao, L. and Dahl, G. (2006) Pannexin 1 in erythrocytes: function without a gap. *Proceedings of the National Academy of Sciences of the United States of America,* 103, 7655-7659.

[96] Lopez, C., Saravia, C., Gomez, A., Hoebeke, J. and Patarroyo, M. A. (2010) Mechanisms of genetically-based resistance to malaria. *Gene,* 467, 1-12.

[97] Low, P. S., Rathinavelu, P. and Harrison, M. L. (1993) Regulation of glycolysis via reversible enzyme binding to the membrane protein, band 3. *The Journal of biological chemistry,* 268, 14627-14631.

[98] Lutz, H. U., Bussolino, F., Flepp, R., Fasler, S., Stammler, P., Kazatchkine, M. D. and Arese, P. (1987) Naturally occurring anti-band-3 antibodies and complement together mediate phagocytosis of oxidatively stressed human erythrocytes. *Proceedings of the National Academy of Sciences of the United States of America,* 84, 7368-7372.

[99] Luzzatto, L., Nwachuku-Jarrett, E. S. and Reddy, S. (1970) Increased sickling of parasitised erythrocytes as mechanism of resistance against malaria in the sickle-cell trait. *Lancet,* 1, 319-321.

[100] Ma, Y. L., Rees, D. C., Gibson, J. S. and Ellory, J. C. (2012) The conductance of red blood cells from sickle cell patients: ion selectivity and inhibitors. *The Journal of physiology,* 590, 2095-2105.

[101] Makhro, A., Hanggi, P., Goede, J. S., Wang, J., Bruggemann, A., Gassmann, M., Schmugge, M., Kaestner, L., Speer, O. and Bogdanova, A. (2013) N-methyl-D-aspartate receptors in human erythroid precursor cells and in circulating red blood cells contribute to the intracellular calcium regulation. *American journal of physiology. Cell physiology,* 305, C1123-1138.

[102] Makhro, A., Wang, J., Vogel, J., Boldyrev, A. A., Gassmann, M., Kaestner, L. and Bogdanova, A. (2010) Functional NMDA receptors in rat erythrocytes. *American journal of physiology. Cell physiology,* 298, C1315-1325.

[103] Malaria Genomic Epidemiology, N. and Malaria Genomic Epidemiology, N. (2014) Reappraisal of known malaria resistance loci in a large multicenter study. *Nature genetics,* 46, 1197-1204.

[104] Manno, S., Takakuwa, Y., Nagao, K. and Mohandas, N. (1995) Modulation of erythrocyte membrane mechanical function by beta-spectrin phosphorylation and dephosphorylation. *The Journal of biological chemistry,* 270, 5659-5665.

[105] Manodori, A. B., Barabino, G. A., Lubin, B. H. and Kuypers, F. A. (2000) Adherence of phosphatidylserine-exposing erythrocytes to endothelial matrix thrombospondin. *Blood,* 95, 1293-1300.

[106] Maria, C., Leonardo, R., Pietro, R., Mario, V., Isabella, V. and Diana, T. (2010) Erythrocytes anion transport and oxidative change in beta-thalassaemias. *Cell biology international,* 34, 655-662.

[107] Matsumoto, Y., Perry, G., Scheibel, L. W. and Aikawa, M. (1987) Role of calmodulin in Plasmodium falciparum: implications for erythrocyte invasion by the merozoite. *European journal of cell biology,* 45, 36-43.

[108] McCurdy, P. R. and Sherman, A. S. (1978) Irreversibly sickled cells and red cell survival in sickle cell anemia: a study with both DF32P and 51CR. *The American journal of medicine,* 64, 253-258.

[109] Melloni, E., Salamino, F., Sparatore, B., Michetti, M. and Pontremoli, S. (1984) Ca2+-dependent neutral proteinase from human erythrocytes: activation by Ca2+ ions and substrate and regulation by the endogenous inhibitor. *Biochemistry international,* 8, 477-489.

[110] Messana, I., Orlando, M., Cassiano, L., Pennacchietti, L., Zuppi, C., Castagnola, M. and Giardina, B. (1996) Human erythrocyte metabolism is modulated by the O2-linked transition of hemoglobin. *FEBS letters,* 390, 25-28.

[111] Mihov, D., Vogel, J., Gassmann, M. and Bogdanova, A. (2009) Erythropoietin activates nitric oxide synthase in murine erythrocytes. *American journal of physiology. Cell physiology,* 297, C378-388.

[112] Mohandas, N. and An, X. (2012) Malaria and human red blood cells. *Medical microbiology and immunology,* 201, 593-598.

[113] Mohandas, N. and Gallagher, P. G. (2008) Red cell membrane: past, present, and future. *Blood,* 112, 3939-3948.

[114] Morelli, A., Grasso, M., Meloni, T., Forteleoni, G., Zocchi, E. and De Flora, A. (1987) Favism: impairment of proteolytic systems in red blood cells. *Blood,* 69, 1753-1758.

[115] Morris, C. R., Kuypers, F. A., Larkin, S., Vichinsky, E. P. and Styles, L. A. (2000) Patterns of arginine and nitric oxide in patients with sickle cell disease with vaso-occlusive crisis and acute chest syndrome. *Journal of pediatric hematology/oncology,* 22, 515-520.

[116] Myssina, S., Huber, S. M., Birka, C., Lang, P. A., Lang, K. S., Friedrich, B., Risler, T., Wieder, T. and Lang, F. (2003) Inhibition of erythrocyte cation channels by erythropoietin. *Journal of the American Society of Nephrology : JASN,* 14, 2750-2757.

[117] Nagababu, E., Fabry, M. E., Nagel, R. L. and Rifkind, J. M. (2008) Heme degradation and oxidative stress in murine models for hemoglobinopathies: thalassemia, sickle cell disease and hemoglobin C disease. *Blood cells, molecules and diseases,* 41, 60-66.

[118] Nguyen, D. B., Wagner-Britz, L., Maia, S., Steffen, P., Wagner, C., Kaestner, L. and Bernhardt, I. (2011) Regulation of phosphatidylserine exposure in red blood cells. *Cellular physiology and biochemistry :*

international journal of experimental cellular physiology, biochemistry, and pharmacology, 28, 847-856.

[119] Olivieri, O., De Franceschi, L., Capellini, M. D., Girelli, D., Corrocher, R. and Brugnara, C. (1994) Oxidative damage and erythrocyte membrane transport abnormalities in thalassemias. *Blood,* 84, 315-320.

[120] Olorunsogo, O. O., Agbolade, F. O., Owojuyigbe, S. O., Adebisi, J. A., Adebayo, A. O. and Okunade, W. G. (1990) Comparative action of calpain on erythrocyte Ca2(+)-pumping ATPase in sickle cell anaemia, essential hypertension and kwashiorkor. *Bioscience reports,* 10, 281-291.

[121] Oonishi, T., Sakashita, K., Ishioka, N., Suematsu, N., Shio, H. and Uyesaka, N. (1998) Production of prostaglandins E1 and E2 by adult human red blood cells. *Prostaglandins and other lipid mediators,* 56, 89-101.

[122] Ortiz, O. E., Lew, V. L. and Bookchin, R. M. (1986) Calcium accumulated by sickle cell anemia red cells does not affect their potassium (86Rb+) flux components. *Blood,* 67, 710-715.

[123] Ortiz, O. E., Lew, V. L. and Bookchin, R. M. (1990) Deoxygenation permeabilizes sickle cell anaemia red cells to magnesium and reverses its gradient in the dense cells. *The Journal of physiology,* 427, 211-226.

[124] Pace, B. S., Shartava, A., Pack-Mabien, A., Mulekar, M., Ardia, A. and Goodman, S. R. (2003) Effects of N-acetylcysteine on dense cell formation in sickle cell disease. *American journal of hematology,* 73, 26-32.

[125] Pauling, L., Itano, H. A. and et al. (1949) Sickle cell anemia a molecular disease. *Science,* 110, 543-548.

[126] Perutz, R. R., Liquori, A. M. and Eirich, F. (1951) X-ray and solubility studies of the haemoglobin of sickle-cell anaemia patients. *Nature,* 167, 929-931.

[127] Peters, L. L., Jindel, H. K., Gwynn, B., Korsgren, C., John, K. M., Lux, S. E., Mohandas, N., Cohen, C. M., Cho, M. R., Golan, D. E. and Brugnara, C. (1999) Mild spherocytosis and altered red cell ion transport in protein 4. 2-null mice. *The Journal of clinical investigation,* 103, 1527-1537.

[128] Platt, O. S., Falcone, J. F. and Lux, S. E. (1985) Molecular defect in the sickle erythrocyte skeleton. Abnormal spectrin binding to sickle inside-our vesicles. *The Journal of clinical investigation,* 75, 266-271.

[129] Puchulu-Campanella, E., Chu, H., Anstee, D. J., Galan, J. A., Tao, W. A. and Low, P. S. (2013) Identification of the components of a glycolytic

enzyme metabolon on the human red blood cell membrane. *The Journal of biological chemistry,* 288, 848-858.

[130] Rank, B. H., Hebbel, R. P. and Carlsson, J. (1984) Oxidation of membrane thiols in sickle erythrocytes. *Progress in clinical and biological research,* 165, 473-477.

[131] Rees, D. C., Williams, T. N. and Gladwin, M. T. (2010) Sickle-cell disease. *Lancet,* 376, 2018-2031.

[132] Rhoda, M. D., Giraud, F., Craescu, C. T. and Beuzard, Y. (1985) Compartmentalization of Ca2+ in sickle cells. *Cell calcium,* 6, 397-411.

[133] Rifkind, J. M., Mohanty, J. G. and Nagababu, E. (2014) The pathophysiology of extracellular hemoglobin associated with enhanced oxidative reactions. *Frontiers in physiology,* 5, 500.

[134] Rodighiero, S., De Simoni, A. and Formenti, A. (2004) The voltage-dependent nonselective cation current in human red blood cells studied by means of whole-cell and nystatin-perforated patch-clamp techniques. *Biochimica et biophysica acta,* 1660, 164-170.

[135] Ronquist, G., Rudolphi, O., Engstrom, I. and Waldenstrom, A. (2001) Familial phosphofructokinase deficiency is associated with a disturbed calcium homeostasis in erythrocytes. *Journal of internal medicine,* 249, 85-95.

[136] Roth, E. F., Jr., Friedman, M., Ueda, Y., Tellez, I., Trager, W. and Nagel, R. L. (1978) Sickling rates of human AS red cells infected in vitro with Plasmodium falciparum malaria. *Science,* 202, 650-652.

[137] Rotter, M. A., Chu, H., Low, P. S. and Ferrone, F. A. (2010) Band 3 catalyzes sickle hemoglobin polymerization. *Biophysical chemistry,* 146, 55-59.

[138] Rubin, E., Schlegel, R. A. and Williamson, P. (1986) Endocytosis in sickle erythrocytes: a mechanism for elevated intracellular Ca2+ levels. *Journal of cellular physiology,* 126, 53-59.

[139] Sabina, R. L., Wandersee, N. J. and Hillery, C. A. (2009) Ca2+-CaM activation of AMP deaminase contributes to adenine nucleotide dysregulation and phosphatidylserine externalization in human sickle erythrocytes. *British journal of haematology,* 144, 434-445.

[140] Schwartz, R. S., Tanaka, Y., Fidler, I. J., Chiu, D. T., Lubin, B. and Schroit, A. J. (1985) Increased adherence of sickled and phosphatidylserine-enriched human erythrocytes to cultured human peripheral blood monocytes. *The Journal of clinical investigation,* 75, 1965-1972.

[141] Scott, M. D., van den Berg, J. J., Repka, T., Rouyer-Fessard, P., Hebbel, R. P., Beuzard, Y. and Lubin, B. H. (1993) Effect of excess alpha-hemoglobin chains on cellular and membrane oxidation in model beta-thalassemic erythrocytes. *The Journal of clinical investigation,* 91, 1706-1712.

[142] Soupene, E., Kemaladewi, D. U. and Kuypers, F. A. (2008) ATP8A1 activity and phosphatidylserine transbilayer movement. *Journal of receptor, ligand and channel research,* 1, 1-10.

[143] Soupene, E. and Kuypers, F. A. (2006) Identification of an erythroid ATP-dependent aminophospholipid transporter. *British journal of haematology,* 133, 436-438.

[144] Steffen, P., Jung, A., Nguyen, D. B., Muller, T., Bernhardt, I., Kaestner, L. and Wagner, C. (2011) Stimulation of human red blood cells leads to Ca2+-mediated intercellular adhesion. *Cell calcium,* 50, 54-61.

[145] Steinberg, M. H., Eaton, J. W., Berger, E., Coleman, M. B. and Oelshlegel, F. J. (1978) Erythrocyte calcium abnormalities and the clinical severity of sickling disorders. *British journal of haematology,* 40, 533-539.

[146] Sugihara, T. and Hebbel, R. P. (1992) Exaggerated cation leak from oxygenated sickle red blood cells during deformation: evidence for a unique leak pathway. *Blood,* 80, 2374-2378.

[147] Sukati, S., Svasti, S., Stifanese, R., Averna, M., Panutdaporn, N., Penglong, T., Melloni, E., Fucharoen, S. and Katzenmeier, G. (2012) Clinical severity of beta-thalassaemia/Hb E disease is associated with differential activities of the calpain-calpastatin proteolytic system. *PloS one,* 7, e37133.

[148] Tanabe, K., Mikkelsen, R. B. and Wallach, D. F. (1982) Calcium transport of Plasmodium chabaudi-infected erythrocytes. *The Journal of cell biology,* 93, 680-684.

[149] Terra, H. T., Saad, M. J., Carvalho, C. R., Vicentin, D. L., Costa, F. F. and Saad, S. T. (1998) Increased tyrosine phosphorylation of band 3 in hemoglobinopathies. *American journal of hematology,* 58, 224-230.

[150] Tiffert, T., Etzion, Z., Bookchin, R. M. and Lew, V. L. (1993) Effects of deoxygenation on active and passive Ca2+ transport and cytoplasmic Ca2+ buffering in normal human red cells. *The Journal of physiology,* 464, 529-544.

[151] Tiffert, T. and Lew, V. L. (1997) Cytoplasmic calcium buffers in intact human red cells. *The Journal of physiology,* 500 (Pt 1), 139-154.

[152] Timmann, C., Thye, T., Vens, M., Evans, J., May, J., Ehmen, C., Sievertsen, J., Muntau, B., Ruge, G., Loag, W., Ansong, D., Antwi, S., Asafo-Adjei, E., Nguah, S. B., Kwakye, K. O., Akoto, A. O., Sylverken, J., Brendel, M., Schuldt, K., Loley, C., Franke, A., Meyer, C. G., Agbenyega, T., Ziegler, A. and Horstmann, R. D. (2012) Genome-wide association study indicates two novel resistance loci for severe malaria. *Nature,* 489, 443-446.

[153] Tsuneshige, A., Imai, K. and Tyuma, I. (1987) The binding of hemoglobin to red cell membrane lowers its oxygen affinity. *Journal of biochemistry,* 101, 695-704.

[154] Vandorpe, D. H., Xu, C., Shmukler, B. E., Otterbein, L. E., Trudel, M., Sachs, F., Gottlieb, P. A., Brugnara, C. and Alper, S. L. (2010) Hypoxia activates a Ca2+-permeable cation conductance sensitive to carbon monoxide and to GsMTx-4 in human and mouse sickle erythrocytes. *PloS one,* 5, e8732.

[155] Wagner, G. M., Chiu, D. T., Yee, M. C. and Lubin, B. H. (1986) Red cell vesiculation--a common membrane physiologic event. *The Journal of laboratory and clinical medicine,* 108, 315-324.

[156] Walder, J. A., Chatterjee, R., Steck, T. L., Low, P. S., Musso, G. F., Kaiser, E. T., Rogers, P. H. and Arnone, A. (1984) The interaction of hemoglobin with the cytoplasmic domain of band 3 of the human erythrocyte membrane. *The Journal of biological chemistry,* 259, 10238-10246.

[157] Wang, J., van Bentum, K., Sester, U. and Kaestner, L. (2014) Calcium homeostasis in red blood cells of dialysis patients in dependence of erythropoietin treatment. *Frontiers in physiology,* 5, 16.

[158] Wasserman, M. (1990) The role of calcium ions in the invasion of Plasmodium falciparum. *Blood cells,* 16, 450-451.

[159] Wasserman, M., Alarcon, C. and Mendoza, P. M. (1982) Effects of Ca++ depletion on the asexual cell cycle of Plasmodium falciparum. *The American journal of tropical medicine and hygiene,* 31, 711-717.

[160] Wasserman, M. and Chaparro, J. (1996) Intraerythrocytic calcium chelators inhibit the invasion of Plasmodium falciparum. *Parasitology research,* 82, 102-107.

[161] Waugh, S. M., Willardson, B. M., Kannan, R., Labotka, R. J. and Low, P. S. (1986) Heinz bodies induce clustering of band 3, glycophorin, and ankyrin in sickle cell erythrocytes. *The Journal of clinical investigation,* 78, 1155-1160.